GOODBYE
SUGAR

Goodbye Sugar

Elsa Jones

GILL & MACMILLAN

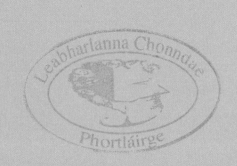

Gill & Macmillan
Hume Avenue
Park West
Dublin 12
www.gillmacmillanbooks.ie

© Elsa Jones 2015

978 0717 1 6689 3

Design by www.grahamthew.com
Photography and food styling by A Fox in
the Kitchen
Edited by Kristin Jensen
Indexed by Adam Pozner
Printed by Printer Trento Srl, Italy

This book is typeset in Gibson.

The paper used in this book comes from the
wood pulp of managed forests. For every tree
felled, at least one tree is planted, thereby
renewing natural resources.

A CIP catalogue record for this book is
available from the British Library.

Acknowledgements

I'm extremely grateful to everyone who has helped make this book a reality.

To my husband, Nick, your endless love and support makes everything possible. Thank you.

To all the team at Gill & Macmillan, thank you for believing in this project and helping me turn a vision into reality; Conor Nagle, Teresa Daly and Catherine Gough, it's been a pleasure working with you.

To Niamh Tyndall and Tara Carey at NK Management, a huge thank you for getting behind me and helping to make this book a success.

A big thanks to Kristin Jensen for the meticulous editing and words of encouragement, and to Graham Thew for putting so much thought and creativity into the book design.

I have Zita and Rob from A Fox in the Kitchen to thank for the gorgeous food photography and styling; we had lots of giggles in my kitchen during the food shoot.

To my family, thank you for your love and thoughtfulness. And finally, to my little boy, Christian, whose cheeky little smile makes everything worthwhile.

CONTENTS

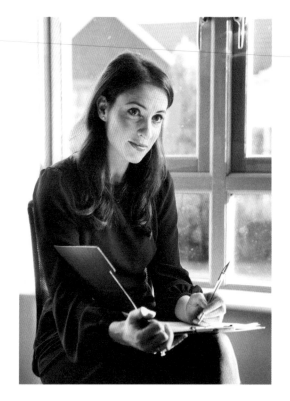

PREFACE

IT'S A WHITE, powdery substance that gives you guaranteed pleasure. The more you have it, the more you want it. You can't get it off your mind, so you keep coming back for more. Even when you try to stay away from it, it finds ways to sneak back into your life every single day and you feel powerless in its presence.

You'd be forgiven for thinking we're talking about some dangerous or illegal drug here, but believe it or not, we're talking about sugar. It may seem harmless in comparison, but it does have similar addictive qualities and it also has the power to wreak havoc on our health. We all know that too much sugar is bad for us, but nowadays we're swamped with the stuff and, as a result, we're hooked.

Over the last few decades sugar has crept into all areas of our daily diet, from the sweet treats we award ourselves to family essentials such as yoghurt, soup and cereal. In fact, it may surprise you to know that the average person consumes over 20 teaspoons per day. The World Health Organization currently recommends that we limit our sugar intake to no more than 6 teaspoons per day. However, sticking to this limit is a lot easier said than done because most of the sugar we consume each day is done unknowingly via everyday 'health foods' that have had sugar added to them.

But why should you care? Is sugar really that bad for you? In a word, yes. It's no secret that too much sugar leads to weight gain, but the effects that sugar has on our bodies go far beyond our waistlines. The sad truth is that many of us are digging our own graves one sweet spoonful at a time.

Research shows that a high-sugar diet can be toxic to the body. It has been linked to the three main killers worldwide: heart disease, cancer and diabetes. A high sugar intake is also linked to fatigue, mood swings, PMS, lowered immunity, digestive problems, premature ageing … the list goes on and on.

Yet despite all the health warnings, many of us have real difficulty resisting our cravings for the sweet stuff, and there are two good reasons why. Firstly, as humans, we are biologically programmed to like sweet foods. When we eat something sugary, it stimulates the release of dopamine in our brain, which makes us feel pleasure. The brain recognises and likes this feeling and begins to crave more, which is how we can become both physically and emotionally dependent on it. In fact, it may frighten you to learn that heroin, morphine and sugar all stimulate the same receptors in our brain.

Secondly, food manufacturers know of our weakness for all things sweet and take full advantage by adding as much sugar as possible to everyday foods, which continually feeds and re-enforces our sweet tooth. It's a vicious cycle and we're easy prey.

And that's just the physical side of things. Sugar has become so entrenched into our everyday lives that many of us have become emotionally dependent on it as well. It's what we reach for to help us cope with the challenges of day-to-day life. It's no wonder so many of us have trouble kicking the sugar habit.

So is it possible to break free from sugar? Yes, it is, provided you get to the real roots of the problem first. *Goodbye Sugar* is here to help you do just that.

INTRODUCTION

IF YOU'RE READING THIS, chances are you've tried to cut down on sweet foods in the past and have realised that it's a hell of a lot easier said than done. You may even feel powerless against your sugar cravings. If you do, let me tell you that you're certainly not alone. I would say that at least two-thirds of my clients tell me they experience strong and persistent cravings for sweet foods on a daily basis. In fact, most say they feel addicted to sugar and cite sugar cravings as their biggest obstacle to losing weight and keeping it off. I'd have to agree. Not only does sugar prevent you from maintaining your ideal weight, it also zaps your energy and mood and keeps you trapped in a cycle of wanting more and more.

But it's not just physical cravings that keep us hooked. Whether you realise it or not, you probably have some strong emotional ties that need to be addressed too. Your attachment to sugar is likely to be deeply ingrained into your day-to-day routine and social practices. It's what you reward yourself with after a hard day's work, how you celebrate special occasions, soothe away negative emotions and how you treat yourself at the weekend. Most of us fall into a sugar habit over time without even realising it. It's an easy habit to make, but a difficult one to break.

Through my consultation work, I have helped countless clients overcome their sugar cravings, lose weight and feel great by giving them targeted dietary advice and a nutrition plan to follow. For some, simply changing their eating habits is enough to kick the sugar habit for good; for others, not so much.

I have found that many clients do really well with dietary changes for a period of time, but as time goes by and real-life obstacles set in, many start falling back into old habits. I wondered why some people would do so well and others wouldn't. And then it hit me. Sugar isn't just *physically* addictive; it's *emotionally* addictive too.

I realised that the dietary advice I was giving was perfectly sound; it's just that for some people it was only addressing one part of the problem: the physical side. To enable clients to overcome their sugar habit for good, I'd need to help them identify and address the psychological and emotional factors behind their eating patterns as well.

To do this, I decided to enhance my skills as a Nutritional Therapist by completing a diploma in cognitive behavioural therapy (CBT), which research shows to be the most widely validated and effective form of psychological therapy available today. In a nutshell, CBT helps people understand the thoughts and feelings that influence all types of behaviour, including eating. Hundreds of studies have demonstrated the effectiveness of CBT for weight management and I have found that using CBT coaching techniques as part of my sessions is extremely effective in helping my clients change their eating habits for good.

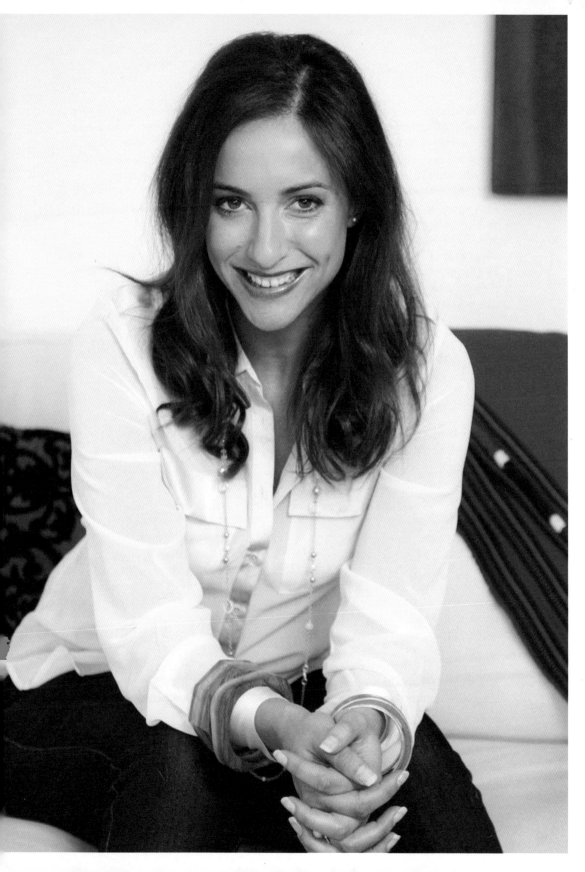

Essentially, I have combined my qualifications and expertise in nutrition with relevant CBT coaching techniques and created an effective two-step programme that combines nutritional science with powerful psychological tools to beat cravings, conquer emotional eating, reframe negative thoughts and ultimately have a controlled and healthy relationship with all types of food – including sugar.

As my success rates rose, I began to think about how I could bring these tools to as many people as possible, and so the idea for *Goodbye Sugar* was born. I want to share my knowledge with you so that you, too, can enjoy the freedom that comes from true health. This is a tried and tested plan that I have created through years of experience working with people who struggle with unhealthy eating habits and weight. Bottom line: it works. I have seen hundreds of clients take back control over their eating habits and their health using the tools I'm about to give you. It's your turn now and I'll be here to guide you every step of the way.

•

Why *Goodbye Sugar* works

YOU MAY HAVE already made several attempts to quit sugar in the past by going on a 'sugar detox' or a 'sugar cleanse'. You probably felt great for a while, but once the novelty wore off and day-to-day problems set in, you went straight back to your old eating habits, right?

There's a reason why sugar detox diets don't work in the long term for a lot of people. It's because they only address a physical dependency on sugar but ignore the emotional stronghold that keeps us hooked. *Goodbye Sugar* contains the missing ingredient lacking in other diet plans. What makes this revolutionary programme different is that it works by not only targeting your physical dependency on sugar, but your emotional dependency too – in other words, the part of you that 'needs' chocolate or biscuits when you're feeling tired, stressed, bored, lonely or just really want some comfort or a treat.

Your physical dependency on sugar will be addressed with a healthy eating plan specifically devised to reset your taste buds, balance your blood sugar and curb your sweet cravings for good. It starts with a **10-Day Sugar Challenge** to help jump start the process and is followed by a nutritionally balanced eating plan full of normal everyday foods that is enjoyable and most importantly, sustainable.

There are no counting calories or points, no shakes or pills and no off-limits food groups, just a practical and satisfying eating plan for life. By focusing on quality protein, healthy fats and good carbohydrates, your body simply won't crave sugar or refined carbohydrates anymore.

However, because the roots of sugar addiction are both physical and emotional, you'll need a combination of physical and psychological approaches to beat it. This is where *Goodbye Sugar* differs from other diet plans. Not only will this book provide you with expert nutrition advice along with a healthy eating plan, it will also teach you powerful psychological tools to break your emotional attachment to sugar.

Using various cognitive behavioural therapy (CBT) techniques, you will learn how to identify and overcome thoughts and behaviours that are sabotaging your health and your weight. You'll also learn essential skills to stay motivated and conquer cravings and emotional eating for good.

The beauty of *Goodbye Sugar* is that it can benefit anyone. It doesn't matter if you have a minor or major weakness for sugar. It makes no difference if you have weight to lose, or not, whether you're male, female, young or old, or whether this is your first or tenth attempt to quit sugar. Everyone can benefit from reducing their sugar intake and this book will give you the tools you need to do it properly.

Practical, hands-on and reader friendly, *Goodbye Sugar* will transform your eating habits by helping you retrain your body and your mind, starting today! Whether you simply want to tame a sweet tooth or break a full-on sugar addiction, *Goodbye Sugar* will help you break your sugar habit gradually and painlessly and ultimately bring your body and mind back into a balanced relationship with sugar.

Are you ready to:

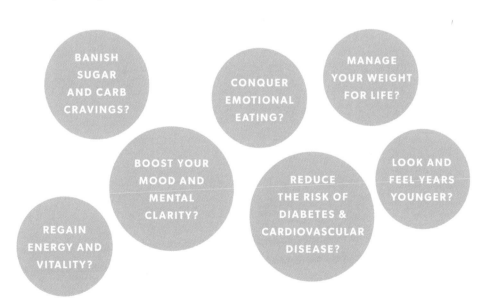

If so, *Goodbye Sugar* is the programme for you!

But before we go any further, let's assess whether you have a healthy relationship with sugar – or not.

Are your sugar cravings out of control?

IT'S NORMAL TO have a craving for something sweet now and again. However, if you're craving sugar and eating sweet foods on a regular basis, it can lead to health and weight problems. Answer yes or no to the questions below to find out if your sugar cravings are beyond the norm.

1 Is a sweet treat part of your everyday routine?

2 Do you think about or crave sweet foods on a daily basis?

3 Do you need caffeine or something sweet to get you going in the morning?

4 Do you often crave refined carbohydrates such as white bread, white pasta, scones and cereals?

5 Do you experience energy slumps throughout the day?

6 Do you feel sleepy after meals?

7 Do you struggle to maintain a healthy weight?

8 Do you need to end a meal with something sweet?

9 Do you have a hard time stopping at a small serving of sweet foods, e.g. two biscuits?

10 Have you ever tried to give up sugar but couldn't stay off it?

11 Do you often turn to sweet foods when you are feeling down, tired or stressed?

If you answered yes to even one of these questions, you are likely to benefit from reading this book. You probably only need to fine tune your existing diet and lifestyle to achieve a health benefit.

If you answered yes to two or more questions, then it's likely that you have an unhealthy relationship with sugar that is affecting your blood sugar balance and hence your everyday health and well-being. If you don't address the underlying causes now, you will continue to struggle with sugar cravings, weight gain, energy slumps and emotional eating.

The good news is that you can reverse the symptoms you are experiencing by following the *Goodbye Sugar* programme and transform the way you look and feel forever.

•

How to use this book

I STRONGLY ADVISE that you read and follow this book in the order that it's written. Each chapter builds on the knowledge gained and the progress made in previous chapters, so you'll get the most out of this programme and progress more effectively if you follow each step in the order set out below.

> **Give yourself at least one week to read and digest Chapters 1 to 5 (inclusive) *before* you embark on the 10-Day Sugar Challenge**

Why the wait? Because you need time to prepare your mindset and your environment. By laying down the groundwork first, you'll be setting yourself up for success.

You'll also need time to reflect on some of the discoveries you'll make about yourself in these chapters and practise the new skills you've learned before you start. Doing so will really stand to you as you embark on the 10-Day Sugar Challenge and means you'll be able to handle any challenges that come your way.

While you are completing the **10-Day Sugar Challenge**, I recommend that you start reading Chapter 6 to familiarise yourself with the principles behind the **Perfect Balance Eating Plan** so that you can seamlessly transfer from one to the other with ease.

Then, in your own time, read Chapters 7 and 8, which will solidify your sugar knowledge and give you the mental and emotional tools you'll need to stay on track and overcome any potential challenges.

Below is an overview of what's to come. I look forward to guiding you on your journey towards better health.

• Chapter 1 •

In Chapter 1 you'll discover how sugar affects your body and your brain, so you'll have a clear understanding of exactly what drives your cravings for sugar and refined carbs and how they can be so addictive. You'll also learn how sugar affects your day-to-day health in terms of weight, energy and mood and you'll gain insight into some of the long-term health effects, such as premature ageing and increased risk of disease.

• Chapter 2 •

Chapter 2 will help you identify whether emotional eating is a factor for you, and if so, to what extent. I'll explain what CBT is, how it works and how it can be used to help change your mindset and your eating habits. We'll also examine whether your thoughts and beliefs about yourself are holding you back, and perhaps for the first time, you'll discover what *truly* motivates you.

• Chapter 3 •

Chapter 3 is all about setting yourself up for success. This is where you'll get organised and prepare your environment *before* you start making any changes to your diet. You'll learn how to create time to succeed and overcome potential challenges. You'll also set realistic and achievable targets for yourself and discover new ways to track your progress.

• Chapter 4 •

Chapter 4 marks the beginning of a new chapter in your life. This is where you'll embark on the 10-Day Sugar Challenge, which allows you to wipe the slate clean and give your body and mind a fresh start. This chapter tells you exactly what you need to do on the 10-Day Sugar Challenge and answers all your practical questions. I'll also provide you with simple meal ideas and helpful supplements for additional support.

• Chapter 5 •

This chapter is designed to help you solve the problems that have made 'dieting' difficult for you in the past. You'll learn the difference between physical and emotional hunger and how you can overcome emotional eating and resist cravings with ease. The mental skills you'll learn in this section will be critical to your long-term success and will help you succeed where other 'diets' have failed.

• Chapter 6 •

You'll be introduced to the Perfect Balance Eating Plan and all it has to offer you. It's important for you to know that this is not a 'diet'. It's simply a guide to adopting healthy eating habits that are practical and sustainable in real life. There's no counting calories or points, no weighing out food, no magic shakes, pills or bars, just normal, everyday foods eaten in moderation.

The Perfect Balance Eating Plan offers guiding principles that will empower you to make healthy choices for yourself and will enable you to live a low-sugar lifestyle with ease. Sticking to the principles will give you the tools to control your cravings, appetite, weight, energy and overall health and well-being.

The meal suggestions and recipes will provide further inspiration as to how you can best apply the principles to your own diet and lifestyle.

• Chapter 7 •

This chapter will ensure you are sugar savvy by teaching you what to look out for on food labels and how to see through marketing jargon. It includes a guide to the best and worst sugar substitutes that are currently on the market. You'll also learn how to thoroughly enjoy eating out, socialising and holidays without going off track.

• Chapter 8 •

The final chapter will help you avoid common diet pitfalls by helping you recognise and challenge negative thoughts and behaviours that may sabotage your progress. You'll learn new thinking skills to overcome 'all or nothing' thinking, feelings of unfairness, mindless eating and how to stop making excuses for yourself. You'll even learn how to fend off 'food pushers' and well-meaning advice givers.

The final section in this chapter offers sound advice on how to deal with possible setbacks, stay on track and most importantly, how to believe that you can succeed as you move forward on your journey towards better health.

So let's get started, shall we?

CHAPTER 1

WHY SUGAR IS ONLY PART OF THE PROBLEM

HOW SUGAR
AFFECTS YOUR
BIOCHEMISTRY

THE NOT-
SO-SWEET
HEALTH EFFECTS

SWEET ADDICTION

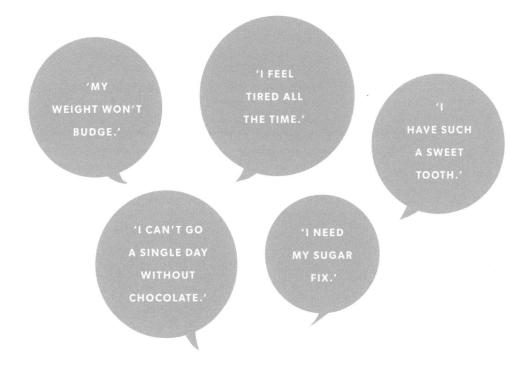

SOUND FAMILIAR? These are the most common phrases I hear from clients who are struggling with their energy levels and weight as a result of their sugar habit.

These statements are usually followed by subsequent admissions of frustration, guilt, shame and helplessness: 'I have no willpower.' 'I don't understand how I can be so disciplined in other areas of my life but not this one.' 'I'm such a pig.' 'I just can't help myself.' 'What's wrong with me?'

If you, too, feel powerless over your eating habits, please know that you're not alone and you can do something about it. The fact that you're reading this book now is testament that you're willing to try something new. Don't waste any more time beating yourself up about it. Instead, invest your energy into taking positive action.

The best way to start is by educating yourself on what exactly is going on in your body. Knowledge is power, and the more understanding you can gain about your reasons for eating the way you do, the more successfully you will be able to combat them.

But before we go any further, I need to make something very clear. When we hear the word *sugar*, we think of the white crystals we spoon into our coffee as well as the obvious high-sugar foods such as chocolate, biscuits, ice cream, cake and sweets. But it's not just sugar itself that causes problems. Certain carbohydrates, which break down into sugar very quickly, cause problems too because they affect our body in a similar way to sugar and can be similarly addictive. These types of carbohydrates are known as **fast-release carbohydrates** and include the likes of white bread, white pasta, refined cereals, crisps, chips and scones.

I cover carbohydrates in detail throughout the book, but for now the main point is this: if you choose to just give up the obvious sources of sugar in your diet, you will look and feel better. However, simply removing the obvious forms of sugar from your diet doesn't go far enough for most people because fast-release carbohydrates act like sugar in the body and thus trigger cravings.

If you continue to eat fast-release carbohydrates, you will remain stuck on the rollercoaster of sugar highs and sugar lows, which means you won't look or feel your best and you'll be in a constant battle with your cravings. On the other hand, if you limit both sugar *and* fast-release carbohydrates, your blood sugar levels will stabilise, which means you'll have much more control over your hunger levels, cravings, weight, energy and mood.

THIS MAY SEEM LIKE A TALL ORDER RIGHT NOW, BUT WITH THE BALANCED DIET AND MINDSET TOOLS I'LL BE GIVING YOU, IT'S 100% DO-ABLE AND PROBABLY A LOT EASIER THAN YOU THINK. FOR NOW, ALL YOU NEED TO DO IS FOLLOW EACH STEP OF THIS BOOK AS IT COMES.

How sugar affects your biochemistry

ONE REALLY IMPORTANT factor in helping someone break a sugar habit is helping them understand the biochemistry that drives their sugar cravings, hunger and addictive pattern of eating. Understanding and taking responsibility for your own personal biochemistry will significantly help you take charge of your cravings and eating habits.

Let's start with the basics in terms of how our bodies break down all types of carbohydrates, not just sugar.

All parts of the body (muscles, brain, heart and liver) need energy to work. This energy comes in the form of glucose (often referred to as sugar, and these terms are used interchangeably). When the stomach digests food, the carbohydrates (sugars and starches) in the food break down into glucose, which is released into the bloodstream.

When blood glucose levels rise, the body (more specifically, the pancreas) responds by producing the hormone insulin. Insulin escorts glucose out of the blood and into the cells, where it can be used for energy. As insulin moves glucose out of the bloodstream and into the cells, blood sugar levels start to drop. Without insulin, blood sugar levels would remain high, which can be very harmful to our health.

Once the glucose is delivered to the cells, three things can happen to it:

1	2	3
It can be used for immediate energy.	It can be converted into a form of glucose known as glycogen and stored in the liver and muscles for later use as a source of energy.	It can be stored as fat. If glycogen stores are already full, then excess glucose is automatically stored as fat.

The amount of glucose and insulin in our bloodstream depends on *when* and *what* we eat as well as *how much*. The rise and fall in insulin and blood sugar is a balancing act and happens many times during the day and night. The aim is to keep your blood sugar levels stable, a balancing act your body is designed to do. In order to maintain blood sugar balance, this mechanism must run efficiently with just the right amount of insulin – not too much and not too little.

• How things go awry •

In healthy people with a *balanced diet*, this mechanism works very well. However, many people, and possibly you, have unknowingly created a set of circumstances that has led your body to lose this balancing act by eating in an *unbalanced way.*

The fact of the matter is that your body's sensitive mechanism for keeping your blood sugar in balance simply cannot cope with the daily onslaught of sugar and fast-release carbohydrates (*and* possibly caffeine and alcohol) that have become part and parcel of our 21st-century diet and lifestyle.

Little by little, the system starts to breaks down. The result is rollercoaster blood sugar levels, which in turn leads to out of control sugar and carb cravings, all of which set the stage for sugar addiction and weight problems.

Let me elaborate. When you eat sugary foods like biscuits, cakes, chocolate, sweets or soft drinks, your blood sugar levels rise rapidly, giving you what's called a 'sugar high'. But remember, it's not just sugary foods that cause problems. Fast-release carbohydrates like white bread, refined cereals, white pasta or white rice have a similar effect in that the body quickly converts them into glucose, so blood glucose levels spike just as they would if you had consumed sugar. The pancreas recognises that blood glucose levels are very high and responds by producing large amounts of insulin in order to get the glucose out of your blood as quickly as possible.

As a result, your blood sugar levels drop quickly, leading to a 'sugar low' or 'sugar crash', which can make you feel tired and low or unable to concentrate and makes you crave more sugar or carbohydrates to perk yourself back up. A mid-morning or mid-afternoon slump is a classic example of this. Meanwhile, insulin levels remain high in the bloodstream, which is bad news for a number of reasons.

The more frequently your blood sugar is raised, the more insulin you produce. The more insulin you produce, the more fat you store. Essentially, having a high insulin level encourages your body to turn food into fat and inhibits the body's breakdown of stored fat. So you can see how a diet high in sugar and fast-release carbs can lead to weight problems.

But there's more. High insulin levels are a contributing factor in another major health issue of our times: insulin resistance. As previously mentioned, every time you eat sugar or fast-release carbs, your blood sugar level spikes. As a result, more and more insulin will need to be produced in order to get the glucose out of your blood and into your cells.

However, over time your cells may start to become deaf (or resistant) to insulin's call and stop opening up to let glucose in. So your body responds by producing more and more insulin in an effort to be heard. The end result is that your cells become *resistant* to insulin, a condition known as insulin resistance. But remember, your body still has to do something with all the glucose whizzing around your system. So where does all the excess glucose go? You guessed it: it gets stored as fat, particularly around the belly area.

Meanwhile, because your cells have not received the energy they need, you feel tired and lethargic and are left craving more sugar and carbs to perk yourself back up. You can see what a vicious cycle it is.

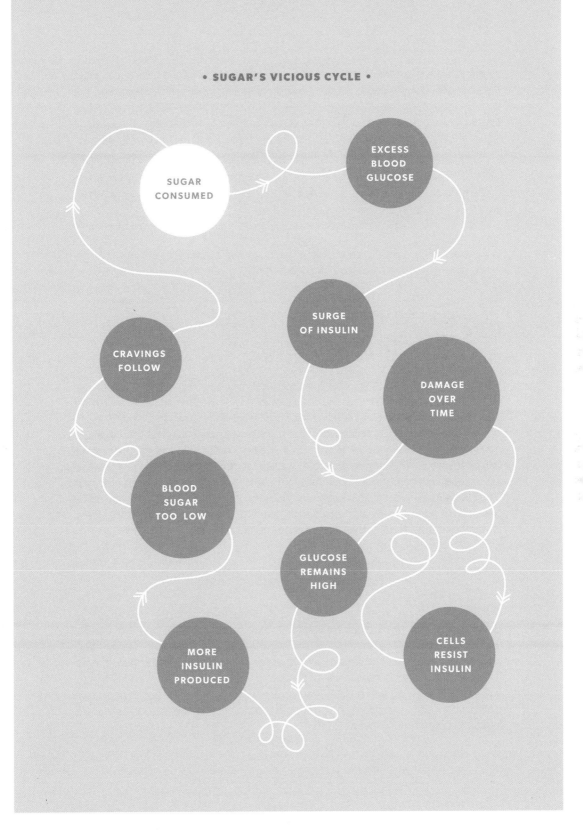

• SUGAR'S VICIOUS CYCLE •

SUGAR CONSUMED

EXCESS BLOOD GLUCOSE

SURGE OF INSULIN

CRAVINGS FOLLOW

DAMAGE OVER TIME

BLOOD SUGAR TOO LOW

GLUCOSE REMAINS HIGH

MORE INSULIN PRODUCED

CELLS RESIST INSULIN

But those are just the short-term effects. If you develop insulin resistance, it can also take you down a slippery road towards diabetes, which is fast becoming the biggest epidemic of the 21st century. Every 10 seconds, a person dies from diabetes-related causes. An estimated 230 million people suffer from diabetes worldwide, a figure the World Health Organization expects to rise to 366 million by 2030.

In the next chapter I'll reveal the full extent to which a high-sugar diet can affect both your short- and long-term health.

•

The not-so-sweet health effects

YOUR PRIMARY MOTIVATION for quitting sugar may be to lose weight, which is a wonderful goal. However, over the course of this book I hope I can make improving your overall health and well-being a major motivation for you too.

Despite numerous warnings by health authorities, I really feel that the vast majority of people are still in denial about just how damaging a high sugar intake can be to our health. Perhaps it's sugar's lack of fat or sodium content or its positive association with celebrations that make it the lesser of evils in people's minds, but if you really knew what all that sugar was doing to your body, you'd probably think twice about adding that extra spoonful of sweetness to your morning cuppa. Here are several unhealthy facts that may surprise you about sugar.

• Sugar drives chronic disease •

Did you know that the amount of sugar you consume directly affects your risk of developing nearly all chronic diseases? This may sound dramatic, but the reasons for this are simple. In a nutshell, excess sugar leads to weight gain. Being overweight or obese majorly increases your chances of developing heart disease, type 2 diabetes and even certain forms of cancer. Of course, the more overweight you are, the higher the impact, but it may surprise you to know that the health risks associated with weighing more than you should start to accumulate as soon as you are as little as seven pounds overweight.

• Sugar has a direct effect on heart disease risk •

If you think that eating fat is the only dietary way to raise your cholesterol levels, think again. When you take in too much sugar, you store the excess amount in your liver in the form of triglycerides, a type of fat that can cling to artery walls as it travels through the bloodstream. High triglyceride levels contribute to atherosclerosis, the formation of plaque in blood vessels. Excess sugar also appears to lower high-density lipoprotein, which is our 'good' cholesterol. Both high cholesterol levels and atherosclerosis increase your risk of developing heart disease.

• Sugar promotes inflammation •

If you're naturally slim, you may think you're off the hook when it comes to weight-related illnesses. However, you don't have to be overweight to be affected by diet-related disease. Every time you spike your blood sugar it promotes inflammation in the body, and inflammation is at the root of pretty much all chronic health conditions, from arthritis and eczema to Alzheimer's, heart disease and stroke.

• The cancer connection •

Most people are still not aware that diet is a primary risk factor for cancer. When the World Cancer Research Fund examined more than 5,000 studies on diet and cancer, they concluded that you could halve your risk of cancer by changing your diet. Eating lots of foods that have sugar added means you are more likely to put on weight. Research categorically shows that being overweight increases your risk of cancer. One reason for this is that excess weight can cause changes in hormone levels. Changes to hormones such as oestrogen or insulin can increase the risk of developing breast, colon or uterine cancer.

• Sugar feeds stress •

Even how we feel on a day-to-day basis can be impacted by sugar consumption. A diet high in sugar and/or fast-release carbohydrates impacts our mood and how we respond to stress because it wreaks havoc on blood sugar balance. If your blood sugar levels are unbalanced, you can end up being trapped in a vicious cycle of sugar highs and sugar lows, which can leave you feeling irritable, moody and constantly craving sugar. If we regularly consume foods that raise our blood sugar levels too quickly, it can throw our hormonal and nervous system out of balance, which can lead to mood swings, feelings of anxiety and poor sleep.

• Sugar suppresses immunity •

If you catch coughs and colds easily, sugar may be the culprit. If you consume excess sugar in your diet, it can greatly reduce your immunity. Studies have shown that an intake of around 35 grams of sugar (about the amount you would find in a can of soft drink or a caramel bar) is enough to cause a 50% reduction in the ability of white blood cells to destroy bacteria.

Research suggests that the immune-suppressing effect of sugar starts less than 30 minutes after ingestion and may last for up to five hours. So if you're consuming sugary foods regularly throughout the day, your immune system may be consistently compromised.

In addition, sugar and artificial sweeteners are anti-nutrients. In other words, they are foods that have no nutritional value but still require nutrients in order to be processed in the body. In effect, they rob us of nutrients. Overconsumption of sugar can cause the body to use up its supplies of important vitamins such as B vitamins and minerals like calcium and magnesium.

• Sugar and ageing •

In terms of our appearance, it's not just our waistlines that are affected. Excess sugar can make your skin dull and speed up the ageing process. At blame is a natural process that's known as glycation, whereby the sugar in your bloodstream attaches to proteins to form harmful new molecules called advanced glycation end products (AGEs for short). The more sugar you eat, the more AGEs you develop. As AGEs accumulate, they damage collagen and elastin, the protein fibres that keep skin firm and elastic.

Once damaged, collagen and elastin become dry and brittle, leading to wrinkles and sagging. These ageing effects start at about age 35 and increase rapidly after that according to a study published in the *British Journal of Dermatology*. In addition, AGEs deactivate your body's natural antioxidant enzymes, leaving your skin more vulnerable to sun damage.

•

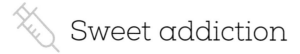 Sweet addiction

There are several ways that sugar causes us to overeat and gain weight and I cover all of these throughout the book. But for the moment, I'm going to focus on the powerful impact sugar has on the reward centres of the brain.

AS HUMANS, WE ARE BIOLOGICALLY
PROGRAMMED TO LIKE SWEET FOODS.
WHEN WE EAT SOMETHING SUGARY, IT
STIMULATES THE RELEASE OF DOPAMINE
IN OUR BRAIN, WHICH MAKES US FEEL
PLEASURE. THE BRAIN RECOGNISES
AND LIKES THIS FEELING AND BEGINS
TO CRAVE MORE. THE HIGH OF A SUGAR
RUSH IS TEMPORARY, THOUGH, AND IS
SWIFTLY FOLLOWED BY A 'SUGAR CRASH',
WHICH CAN LEAVE US FEELING TIRED,
LOW AND CRAVING YET MORE SUGAR.

1. YOU EAT SUGAR
• You like it, you crave it
• It has addictive properties

2. BLOOD SUGAR LEVELS SPIKE
• Dopamine is released in the brain = addiction
• Mass insulin secreted to drop blood sugar levels

3. BLOOD SUGAR LEVELS FALL RAPIDLY
• High insulin levels promote fat storage
• Body craves the lost sugar 'high'

4. HUNGER & CRAVINGS
• Low blood sugar levels cause increased appetite and cravings
• Thus the cycle is repeated

And yet the more sugar you consume, the higher your tolerance becomes, so you need more to get the same effect. This is because the more you over-stimulate the release of dopamine, the more insensitive you become to its effects, so you will need more sugar the next time in order to get the same level of reward.

Due to their powerful effects on the reward centres of the brain, sugar and fast-release carbohydrates function in a somewhat similar way to stimulatory drugs like alcohol, caffeine, nicotine and cocaine. The exact same brain centres are at play.

Of course, that's not to say that everyone who eats sugar will become addicted to it, but sugar certainly does possess addictive qualities that make it easy to become both physically and emotionally dependent on it. And given that it's so readily available, socially acceptable and entrenched into our daily lives, it's a very easy trap to fall into.

We've already explored the physical side of a sugar habit. Now it's time to explore the emotional side of things. In the next chapter, you'll learn how your thoughts, feelings and emotions feed your sugar habit and what you can do about it.

Chocolate is treble trouble:
sugar + stimulants + fat

If you can't go a day without chocolate, there's a good reason why. Of all the sugary foods, chocolate appears to be the most addictive, which is probably why it has become an everyday treat in the Western world.

Not only does it contain high amounts of sugar, it also provides significant quantities of the stimulant theobromine, which gives you a bit of a lift and stimulates serotonin (the happy hormone) production. Chocolate also contains small amounts of caffeine. With its array of sugar, stimulants and fat combined with that melt-in-your-mouth feeling, it's no wonder the world is filled with chocoholics!

CHAPTER 2

ARE YOU AN EMOTIONAL EATER?

ARE YOU
EMOTIONALLY
DEPENDANT
ON SUGAR?

INTRODUCING
CBT: HOW IT
WORKS AND
WHAT IT WILL
DO FOR YOU

IS YOUR
DIET HISTORY
HOLDING YOU
BACK?

ARE YOU
READY AND
WILLING TO
CHANGE?

WHAT *TRULY*
MOTIVATES
YOU?

Are you emotionally dependant on sugar?

IN CHAPTER 1, we learned how sugar affects our bodies and creates physical cravings that keep us hooked. But it's not just biological triggers that influence our eating patterns. There are various other triggers that influence the type of foods we choose and how much we eat.

You're probably most aware of **environmental triggers**, such as seeing or smelling food, like walking through the bakery section of a supermarket and seeing and smelling freshly baked goods. You can also experience **mental triggers** – thinking about or imagining yourself eating a particular food, such as recalling something you enjoyed eating and imagining eating it again or reading a description of food. There are also **social triggers** – particular people or places that encourage you to eat certain foods. For example, you may associate eating popcorn with the cinema or eating cake with a birthday party.

And then there are the biggest triggers of all: **emotional triggers**. These are usually unpleasant or uncomfortable feelings such as stress, tiredness, anger, frustration, sadness, boredom or loneliness. Eating in response to emotional triggers is known as **emotional eating**. Essentially you eat to comfort, suppress or distract yourself from how you are feeling. This can be done consciously or unconsciously.

However, emotional eating can be linked to *positive* feelings too, such as reward, celebration or romance, such as rewarding yourself with tea and biscuits after completing a task or overindulging in a restaurant in an effort to enhance your enjoyment. If you're enjoying eating something, you might eat past the point of fullness because you don't want the feelings of enjoyment to end and so you keep eating in an effort to keep that good feeling going. These are all forms of emotional eating.

• How common is emotional eating? •

Research suggests that 75% of overeating is caused by emotions. From personal experience and from the many years I've counselled people on their eating habits, I'd have to concur. In fact, I've come to understand that we each have our own unique relationship with food that is built up over many years, and like all relationships, sometimes it can be very complicated indeed.

• Why is emotional eating a problem? •

Emotional eating can seriously sabotage your weight and your health because firstly, it causes us to overeat, and secondly, when we emotional eat, it's usually with unhealthy foods.

HOW OFTEN DO YOU REACH
FOR AN APPLE WHEN YOU'RE
LOOKING FOR COMFORT?
MORE OFTEN THAN NOT, WE
TURN TO SUGARY FOODS LIKE
CHOCOLATE, BISCUITS, CAKE
AND ICE CREAM AND/OR FAST-
RELEASE CARBS LIKE BREAD,
SCONES, CHIPS OR CRISPS.

For some, emotional eating can also lead to a vicious cycle. Your emotions trigger you to overeat, you feel guilty, ashamed and frustrated with yourself, and you overeat again to suppress those uncomfortable feelings. I see so many people trapped in the cycle of emotional eating, which is why I believe that getting a handle on any tendency to eat in response to emotions is essential if you want to manage your weight and your health for life.

To date, CBT has proven to be the most successful psychological approach available to combat emotional eating. It helps you understand the triggers behind your emotional eating and changes the way you think and behave around all types of food, including sugar.

In the next section I will explain exactly what CBT is and we'll deal with emotional eating in a lot more detail in Chapter 5. But for now, let's see to what extent your emotions are influencing your eating behaviour. Complete the questionnaire below to gain some insight.

Are You an Emotional Eater?
How often do you eat unhealthy foods or overeat when...

1. You're feeling down or browned off
    (a) Often   (b) Rarely

2. You're trying to postpone doing something you don't feel like doing
    (a) Often   (b) Rarely

3. You're tired and need a pick-me-up
    (a) Often   (b) Rarely

4. You feel stressed or frustrated
    (a) Often   (b) Rarely

5. You're bored and can't think of anything better to do
    (a) Often   (b) Rarely

6. To reward yourself
    (a) Often   (b) Rarely

7. **How often do you eat past the point of just feeling mildly full?**
   (a) Often   (b) Rarely

8. **How often do you experience a *sudden* craving for a specific food, e.g. chocolate?**
   (a) Often   (b) Rarely

9. **How often do you go out of your way to satisfy a particular food craving?**
   (a) Often   (b) Rarely

10. **How often do you feel secretive or guilty in relation to what and how much you ate?**
    (a) Often   (b) Rarely

Mostly **As**

If you answered mostly As then it's likely that emotional eating is an underlying factor in your eating behaviour and needs to be addressed. The good news is that you can take steps to regain control over your eating habits, and the tools in this book will show you how.

Mostly **Bs**

Your eating behaviour does not appear to be strongly linked to your emotions. The tools in this book will help you get a better understanding of what influences your eating behaviour so you can gain more control over your eating habits. It's possible that your eating patterns may be more linked to physiological triggers, which are addressed as part of the 10-Day Sugar Challenge and the Perfect Balance Eating Plan.

Introducing CBT: How it works and what it will do for you

IF YOU'VE STRUGGLED to take control over your eating habits in the past, you've probably beaten yourself up and concluded that you are weak or greedy and don't have any willpower. These things may be a factor, but what's more likely is that you just didn't have the tools you needed to successfully manage your eating habits. The good news is that the techniques involved in cognitive behavioural therapy (CBT) will help you succeed where other diets have failed.

As previously mentioned, many of the psychological tools in *Goodbye Sugar* are based on the principles of CBT. Research has shown cognitive behavioural therapy to be the most widely validated and effective form of psychology therapy today. CBT can be practised in many ways: it can be done individually with a therapist or within a group or it can be done using a self-help book or online programme.

In a nutshell, CBT helps people understand the thoughts and feelings that influence behaviours. It's based on the concept that the way people think affects how they feel and what they do.

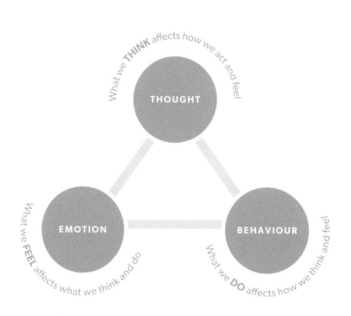

Hundreds of research studies have demonstrated that CBT helps people with a wide range of challenges, including weight management, depression, anxiety, phobias, addictions, obesity and eating disorders. In terms of weight management, it has been shown that combining CBT with lifestyle changes is more effective for long-term weight management than making lifestyle changes alone.

The key element of CBT is that it helps you understand the link between your thoughts, feelings, body and behaviour – in other words, how our behaviours (such as eating) are closely connected to the way we think (our thoughts), our feelings (emotions) and our body (physical reactions). The example below illustrates this.

Mind–body connection

A thought:
'I'll never lose weight because I have no willpower. I've tried and failed so many times before, so what's the point?
Which is connected to …

A feeling:
Feeling defeated and hopeless
Which is connected to …

A physical feeling:
Lethargic, no energy and craving sugar, e.g. chocolate
Which is connected to …

Behaviour:
Overindulging on chocolate to comfort yourself

I truly believe that to consistently eat in a controlled, balanced and healthy way, you need to make permanent changes in your thinking. *Goodbye Sugar* will help you to recognise and challenge negative or sabotaging thoughts or beliefs, such as 'I have no willpower', 'I don't have time for this' or 'It's just too hard' that hold you back.

In the past, you may have been able to make short-term changes to your eating habits and got some short-term results. During the first few weeks, you may find it relatively easy to make changes and feel on a high.

But bit by bit, the novelty wears off and it starts getting more difficult. Real-life challenges set in: your schedule gets busy, you feel tired, stressed or emotional, you attend a social event, you go on holidays, temptation abounds and you start having cravings. And you probably find yourself coming up with any number of reasons to stray from your diet:

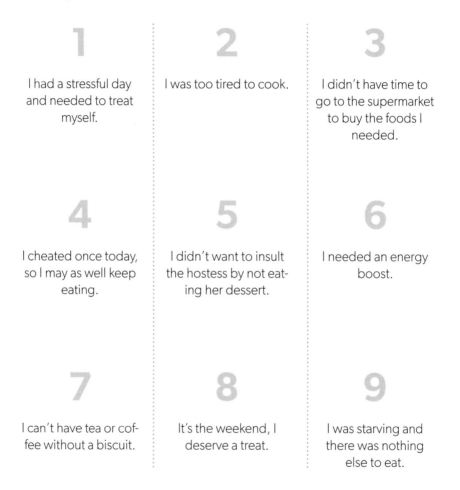

1 I had a stressful day and needed to treat myself.

2 I was too tired to cook.

3 I didn't have time to go to the supermarket to buy the foods I needed.

4 I cheated once today, so I may as well keep eating.

5 I didn't want to insult the hostess by not eating her dessert.

6 I needed an energy boost.

7 I can't have tea or coffee without a biscuit.

8 It's the weekend, I deserve a treat.

9 I was starving and there was nothing else to eat.

Using the set of psychological strategies in this book, you will learn how to resist temptation when you're confronted with a variety of different challenges, including cravings, stress, tiredness, lack of motivation, feelings of deprivation and social pressure. These strategies will take practice at first, but over time they'll become automatic for you and will be the key to your long-term success.

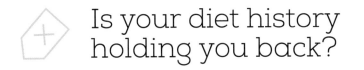

Is your diet history holding you back?

'INSANITY: DOING THE SAME THING OVER AND OVER AGAIN AND EXPECTING DIFFERENT RESULTS.'

ALBERT EINSTEIN

CAN YOU RELATE to any of the following experiences and/or thoughts and feelings?

- You begin a new diet and are filled with confidence and enthusiasm that *this* is going to be THE ONE that will finally work for you. Then you eat something you shouldn't, feel really guilty and ashamed that you 'broke the diet' and have 'failed' yet again, and now you can't seem to work up the enthusiasm and willpower to start again.

- Every diet you've tried in the past worked for a while, but eventually you gained all the weight back and more. When you think of all of the sacrifices you've made on previous diets and all of the time, effort and money you've put in, not to mention the emotional highs and lows you've experienced, you can't help but look back and feel angry and upset that the only lasting result was a feeling of failure and disappointment.

- What's worse is that after all that, you are still desperate to find a solution but feel too defeated and hopeless to try yet another diet or eating plan. You think, 'What's the point in trying if I'm just going to fail anyway?'

- And then you may wonder, 'What must others think of me?' You possibly feel that you've let family or loved ones down. You're probably thinking that everyone is judging you and thinks that you are weak or greedy or a failure. You can't bear the thought of them seeing you try and fail again. It's just too embarrassing.

If you can relate to any of the above, then there is a good chance that your thoughts and feelings about your own diet history have led you to develop certain beliefs about yourself that won't serve you going forward. 'I've no willpower' is a common belief many people hold. 'I'm a failure' is another one.

The flow chart below shows how negative thoughts or beliefs prompt negative feelings, which prompt negative action or inaction.

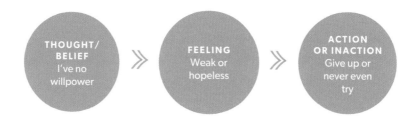

I want you to think about **what has held you back** in the past and **how it made you feel** about yourself, because it may have a lot to do with where you are now. It can be useful to write your thoughts and observations down. You may do so in the space provided below or in a private journal, whatever works.

_____

_____

_____

_____

_____

_____

_____

_____

_____

_____

_____

_____

Over the course of this book, you're going to learn how to recognise negative thoughts and beliefs that may be holding you back. You'll learn how to challenge them and reframe them into more positive, empowering ones. Keep a journal and record negative or self-defeating thoughts as they pop into your head. Over time, you'll start to see common thinking patterns emerge. Overleaf is an example of how to reframe a negative thought (based on beliefs from past failures) into a more positive, helpful one.

What are you thinking?

Negative, unhelpful thought:

I'll fail eventually, so what's the point?

Positive, helpful thought:

I don't have a crystal ball, so I don't know whether or not this will work for me. The one thing I do know for sure is that I haven't used all of the tools in this book before. I want things to change, so I am willing to try something different.

As time goes by you'll probably have lots of sabotaging thoughts, which is to be expected. Throughout this book, I'll show you how to apply this reframing method to a variety of negative thoughts that might otherwise hinder your progress. My clients tell me over and over again how this reframing method makes a big difference to their mindset. It works for them and it will work for you too. It just takes a little practice.

When you're reframing negative thoughts into more positive, helpful ones, it's important that you use wording that *you* really connect with. My wording is only there to inspire and guide you in the right direction, but it's important that you adjust them to suit your own personal thoughts and beliefs. It can be useful to write a helpful response to a negative thought so that you can refer to it the next time it comes up.

The purpose of reminding you of past failures is not to make you feel bad about yourself. What I'm trying to get across is that if you're carrying around negative emotional or psychological baggage based on previous diet failures, it could sabotage your future efforts if you let it. The good news is that even just being *aware* of them is the first step towards letting go of thoughts and beliefs that no longer serve you.

Another reason why I've asked you to look back on your diet history is to remind you that whatever you've tried in the past didn't work for you or simply wasn't enough. If it had been, you'd now be fully in control of your eating and would look and feel your best. So if you're tempted to skip some of the steps on this programme, remind yourself that not using these techniques in the past hasn't got you to where you want to be.

Bottom line: If you want things to change, you need to do something different.

Are you ready and willing to change?

How satisfied are you with your current eating habits?

NOT AT ALL ❏   A MODERATE AMOUNT ❏   COMPLETELY ❏

How satisfied are you with your current weight?

NOT AT ALL ❏   A MODERATE AMOUNT ❏   COMPLETELY ❏

How willing are you to change your eating habits?

NOT AT ALL ❏   A MODERATE AMOUNT ❏   COMPLETELY ❏

How willing are you to put in the time needed to shop for foods listed on your nutrition plan and prepare and cook healthy meals?

NOT AT ALL ❏   A MODERATE AMOUNT ❏   COMPLETELY ❏

How willing are you to make sacrifices to achieve your health goals?

NOT AT ALL ❏   A MODERATE AMOUNT ❏   COMPLETELY ❏

Making changes to your diet and lifestyle can be challenging on a number of levels. You may find yourself resisting some of the changes that are coming your way, which is perfectly normal, yet counterproductive. The reason I asked the previous questions is because if you don't feel fully prepared to make the changes that are necessary in order to achieve your goals, then you will need to learn how to increase your motivation factors, because these changes are essential.

Wanting to change is not enough. You need to be willing to do what is necessary to bring about change. This may involve making sacrifices and withstanding uncomfortable feelings along the way. The more motivated you are, the more likely you'll be willing to make these changes and sacrifices. This is why it's so important that you figure out what *truly* motivates you.

Can you recall a time in your life when you successfully made a change for the better? If so, what motivated you to do so? *Goodbye Sugar* will help you find your true motivating factors and teach you how to maintain your motivation levels as you go through the process of change.

Remember, change requires change.

Before we go any further, take a moment to consider this: where will your health and weight be a year from now if nothing changes?

•

What *truly* motivates you?

I'M SURE YOU have many reasons why you want to reduce your sugar intake and improve your diet. You could probably list a handful of them right now. But if you're like most people who have a weakness for sugar, you don't automatically think of all these reasons when you're craving something sweet. In fact, they're possibly the farthest things from your mind when you're focused on what you're eating or about to eat.

One essential technique that will help you control your eating is to *continually* remind yourself of what you will *gain* by reducing your sugar intake and living a low-sugar lifestyle. If you *continually* focus on what you are gaining, you'll be a lot less likely to get swept away by cravings or feel deprived in any way.

The most effective way of doing this is to write down all the reasons why you want to live a low-sugar lifestyle and put it somewhere where you can read it every single day. It's crucial for you to remind yourself of the benefits again and again, even when you're not craving or feeling tempted. If the benefits are always at the forefront of your mind, you'll be much more likely to resist temptation when it strikes.

• Motivational exercise •

This is a simple exercise, but a crucial one for laying down foundations for your success. All you need to do is write down all of the benefits you will receive by reducing your sugar intake and following a healthy diet. The action of writing them down will help you clarify exactly what your goals are and cement them in your brain.

Remember, dietary changes are likely to have a knock-on effect on many aspects of your health and well-being, both now and in the future, including your **weight, energy levels, stamina, mood, mental clarity, confidence, skin, sleep, digestion and heart health,** to name just a few. These in turn will have positive effects on all aspects of your daily life, including **family life, relationships, work, social life, health risks, fitness, etc.**

If you ask yourself the following questions, it will help you recognise all you stand to gain by changing your diet.

How will it affect my weight?

How will I look?

What will I wear?

How will it benefit my current health?

How will it safeguard my health in the future?

What will I do when I have more energy?

How will it change my mood?

How will others view me?

How will I feel about myself?

How will it affect my family?

What will change at work?

How will my relationships change?

What will I do that I wouldn't do before?

What activities or hobbies will I take up?

Below are some examples of benefit lists that my clients have made. You'll see that a lot of the benefits they've listed are those that arise as a result of weight loss and an improvement in energy and well-being. They've listed both short- and longer-term benefits of being slim and healthy, which is extra motivating.

BENEFITS LIST, Susan, 42

I'll have more energy to play with my daughter.

I'll feel good about cooking healthy meals for my family and setting a good example.

I'll have the confidence to get into the pool with my daughter when I take her swimming.

I'll enjoy being photographed and finally get a family portrait done.

I'll be able to wear a nice dress to my daughter's Communion.

I'll be at less risk of developing type 2 diabetes, like my mother.

I'll feel in control.

I'll enjoy physical intimacy more.

I'll enjoy wearing skirts with bare legs this summer.

I'll feel like me again.

BENEFITS LIST, Emma, 28

I'll be able to wear skinny jeans.

I'll enjoy shopping and trying on clothes.

I'll enjoy dancing again.

I'll be able to wear a bikini on holidays.

I won't feel judged by my weight.

I'll feel comfortable in my work skirt.

I'll feel more alert and focused at work.

My skin will be clear and bright.

I'll have the confidence to start dating again.

I'll enjoy being a bridesmaid at my sister's wedding.

I'll like myself better.

My parents will be proud of me.

BENEFITS LIST, Sean, 48

My cholesterol will come down along with my weight, so I won't have to take medication.

I'll feel more in control over my current and future health.

My digestion will be better, with less reflux and indigestion.

I'll feel more assertive at work and more confident giving presentations.

I'll be more likely to go for that promotion.

I'll have more energy and mobility on the golf course.

I'll be in better form with my family.

I'll be able to keep up with my sons in the park.

I'll be in a better position to manage my stress levels.

I'll sleep better.

Now it's your turn to create your own benefits list. What will *you* gain?

1. _____
   _____
   _____

2. _____
   _____
   _____

3. _____
   _____
   _____

4. _____
   _____
   _____

5. _____
   _____
   _____

6. _____
   _____
   _____

7. _____
   _____
   _____

8. _____
   _____
   _____

9. _____
   _____
   _____

10. _____
    _____
    _____

• Helpful hints •

If you would prefer not to write in the book, you can just use a pen and paper. Put the list somewhere you will see it every day, like the inside of your wardrobe door or on the inside cover of your diary.

If you prefer not to use paper or you want to keep your list private, you could transfer your benefits list onto your smartphone or computer and perhaps even set yourself a reminder to look at them daily.

Decide *when* exactly you plan to read your benefits list. **For the next six weeks, I recommend reading it at least once per day, but ideally more than that**. You might find it helpful to read it right before every meal, for example. You should also schedule a reminder to read it at your trigger times, i.e. those moments of the day when you're likely to succumb to cravings.

What are you thinking?

Are you having negative or resistant thoughts about doing this motivational exercise? If so, reframe your thoughts into more positive, helpful ones. Here's an example.

Negative, unhelpful thought:
I don't need to remind myself of the reasons why I want to quit sugar. I know them.

Positive, helpful thought:
But when I'm craving, my mind is focused on the food, not on my weight or my health. That's why I have to keep all of the benefits at the forefront of my mind so that they'll be there when temptation strikes.

CHAPTER 3

SETTING TARGETS AND TRACKING PROGRESS

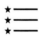

HOW TO
MEASURE
YOUR
PROGRESS

SET
YOURSELF UP
FOR SUCCESS

How to measure your progress

EVERYBODY HAS DIFFERENT reasons why they want to reduce their sugar intake and improve their diet. Now that you've completed your **benefits list** (page 26), you should have a clear vision of what exactly it is you want to get out of this lifestyle change. You may have lots of general reasons or just one very specific reason.

For example, you may want to lose weight and have more energy or you may want to improve your digestion, lower your cholesterol or even prevent diabetes. Perhaps you want to achieve all of the above and more. It's entirely achievable, because as previously mentioned, changing your diet often has a knock-on effect on all aspects of health and well-being. I see evidence of this every day in my work as a nutritionist.

Whatever *your* reasons are, it's important that you set realistic targets for yourself and have ways of tracking your progress. In order to be able to measure results, you need to assess where you are now so that you have an accurate starting point. There are several ways to do this. Some or all may be relevant to you.

• Weight •

If your goal is to lose weight, weigh yourself before embarking on the 10-Day Sugar Challenge. Ideally weigh yourself undressed, first thing in the morning, and stick to weighing yourself in the same condition each time thereafter.

I strongly urge you to avoid weighing yourself *during* the 10-Day Sugar Challenge. You can do so afterwards if you wish. While a large percentage of participants do report weight loss after the 10-Day Sugar Challenge, it isn't the main focus of the programme, nor is it the only indicator of whether or not the programme is working for you. A boost in energy and mood and a reduction in cravings are actually better indicators of progress.

Your primary motivation for quitting sugar may be to lose weight, which is a fantastic goal to have. However, I encourage you not to make weight loss your *only* goal. Otherwise, if you have a week where you don't get the weight loss results you expected for whatever reason, you'll feel deflated and de-motivated. If you only focus on weight loss, it will make you blind to all the other health benefits this programme has to offer, such as increased energy, better mood and sleep, improved digestion as well as a reduced risk of developing diet-related illnesses such as heart disease and diabetes.

WHAT RESULTS CAN I EXPECT?

If you are carrying extra weight, it's likely that you will lose weight at a steady pace by following the eating plan as set out in the **10-Day Sugar Challenge** and thereafter on the **Perfect Balance Eating Plan**. The average weight loss I've observed amongst clients is 1–2lb per week, which is a healthy rate to lose weight. However, this varies according to many different factors, including how much weight you have to lose, your previous diet history and whether or not you have any hormonal imbalances or thyroid issues. Some people lose weight fast, others slower. Remember, this is not a 'quick fix' diet, it's an eating plan for life, so slow and sustainable results are what we're after.

ALTERNATIVE WAYS TO MEASURE WEIGHT LOSS

Don't get too hung up on numbers on a scale. Weigh yourself once per week *if* you find it motivating to do so. Some do, whereas others prefer to use their clothes as an indicator of weight loss. You don't need a scale to prove you've lost weight if you can now fit into a pair of jeans that you previously couldn't get past your hips!

There are plenty of ways to measure weight loss beyond the scale, so don't rely on it as the only way of tracking your progress. Your local gym, health centre, GP or pharmacy may offer a service for measuring your body fat percentage using callipers or testing equipment. Aim to reduce your body fat percentage by 1% each month until you fall within a healthy range for your gender and age.

Taking measurements is another way of tracking progress. To ensure accuracy, measure in exactly the same place and with the same type of clothes each time. Here are some tips to help you.

1	2	3
Bust	**Waist**	**Hips**
Place the tape measure across your nipples and measure around the largest part of your chest. Keep the tape parallel to the floor.	Your natural waist lies 1–2 inches above your belly button. Try placing two fingers above your belly button and measure there. When measuring your waist, exhale and measure before inhaling again.	Place the tape measure across the widest part of your hips/buttocks and measure all the way around while keeping the tape parallel to the floor. The fullest part of your hips generally lies 8 inches below your natural waist.

How do you measure up?

A waist measurement greater than 32 inches in adult women and 37 inches in adult men is an indicator that excess fat is being stored around vital organs such as the kidneys, liver and heart. Carrying fat around your middle is linked to many chronic diseases, such as heart disease, diabetes and cancer.

• Blood tests •

If you have particular health concerns, it can be useful to have some blood work done before you embark on your new eating plan and then again three months later to see if the change in diet has made an impact. This is particularly relevant if you have concerns about your cholesterol and/or if you have elevated blood glucose levels.

I have seen many clients achieve a significant drop in their cholesterol levels and a return to normal glucose levels within three months of following the eating plans outlined in this book. Nothing is more motivating than getting a positive before-and-after result, and blood tests provide a tangible way of measuring how well your body is responding to dietary change. Have a chat with your GP if you'd like to have some blood tests done. If you are overweight, you should have your cholesterol and blood glucose levels checked on a regular basis anyway.

• Symptom analysis •

Another excellent way to track your progress is through symptom analysis. The questionnaire below is designed to assess how stable your blood sugar levels are. If you experience some of the symptoms below, it's likely that poor blood sugar control is a factor for you and needs to be addressed. The diet advice in this book will do this for you.

You should fill out this questionnaire now, before you embark on any dietary changes, and then again about six weeks from now to see if your score is different. I'm willing to bet you'll see a significant improvement after four weeks or less.

Blood sugar balance and wellness assessment

Circle your answers and add up your total score.
0 = Never   1 = Sometimes   2 = Often

I still feel tired 20 minutes after rising in the morning.
0 / 1 / 2

I need caffeine and/or something sweet like toast with jam to give me a kick start in the morning.
0 / 1 / 2

I crave sweet foods and/or refined carbs like bread, scones or pasta.
0 / 1 / 2

I struggle to stay at my ideal weight.
0 / 1 / 2

I feel too tired to exercise.
0 / 1 / 2

I have energy slumps and/or difficulty concentrating in the afternoons.
0 / 1 / 2

I crave something sweet like chocolate after meals and/or I feel sleepy after meals.
0 / 1 / 2

I have mood swings.
0 / 1 / 2

I get dizzy or irritable coming up to mealtimes.
0 / 1 / 2

I get stressed easily.
0 / 1 / 2

Score

0-4 Your blood sugar balance is likely to be relatively good. You probably only need to tweak your existing diet and habits to experience a health benefit. The advice in this book will help you do this easily.

5-9 You are starting to experience some symptoms of imbalanced blood sugar. If you follow the diet advice in this book, you should soon start to feel a significant improvement in your symptoms.

10-14 It's likely that you are struggling with poor blood sugar balance. You need to address the underlying causes now, otherwise you will continue to experience symptoms such as sugar cravings, weight gain, energy slumps and poor concentration.

15 or more Your blood sugar balance appears to be out of control and your health may be at risk. I encourage you to take action now. It's likely that you are caught in a vicious cycle of sugar highs and sugar lows, but you can break this cycle and reverse the symptoms you are experiencing by following the diet advice in this book. You will feel and look so much better as your body starts to restore its own natural balance.

•

Set yourself up for success

Wanting to change is not the same as being ready to change.

I'm a big believer in the saying 'if you fail to plan, you plan to fail'. In order to be successful with this programme, you will first need to set yourself up for success. In practical terms, this means taking a few days or even up to a week to get yourself organised and prepare your environment before you start the 10-Day Sugar Challenge.

It's wise to have a think about what potential obstacles and challenges may come your way as you embark on your new eating plan. I like to think of it as advance trouble-shooting. When you identify potential obstacles, it gives you the power to anticipate them and plan how you're going to handle them so that you aren't tempted to give up when you hit your first hurdle. Anticipating and planning for potential obstacles empowers you to succeed. Here are several steps that will help you do just that.

• Remove temptation •

Limit your exposure to trigger foods when you're starting out. Over time, with the tools in this book, you will have fewer cravings and will develop the skills to resist temptation, but 'out of sight, out of mind' is a good policy for now.

As such, go through all your food cabinets, fridge and freezer, and if possible, give away or else throw out foods that are not on your food plan and/or foods that are personally tempting for you, i.e. the foods you reach for when you're feeling emotional, tired, etc. If they're not there, you can't eat them!

Don't feel guilty about throwing out unhealthy food. It's going to be wasted one way or the other, either in the rubbish bin or in your body, where it will get stored as fat – which would you rather it be? If this isn't possible because of other members of your household, move these foods to a high shelf or to the back of the fridge or cupboard.

• Ask for support •

If you share your kitchen with others at home or at work, ask them for their co-oper-ation and support in helping to keep tempting foods out of your sight as much as possible, particularly at the start. Rather than demanding that they also make changes, phrase your request in a nice way, such as 'Would you be willing to help me by...?', 'Could we come to some agreement whereby...?'

For example, when Susan started her eating plan she made a 'no sweets in the house' rule for the whole family. However, as a compromise she agreed that once a week her husband would take the kids to the shop and they could choose one serving of whatever sweets they wanted as a treat. That way the kids learned that sweets are not an everyday food and Susan was removed from all temptation.

• Start weaning yourself off stimulants •

In the days leading up to your sugar challenge, start to slowly wean yourself off sugar and caffeine to ease the withdrawal process. On the 10-Day Sugar Challenge, I recommend eliminating or at least reducing your caffeine intake. Going cold turkey on both of these addictive substances at the same time can be tough, but weaning yourself slowly will ease this process. In the week leading up to the 10-Day Sugar Challenge, start by having only half your regular consumption, then cutting that half in half for a few days and so on.

• Plan your meals in advance •

When you've finished this chpater, have a good look at the list of foods on the 10-Day Sugar Challenge and tick the foods that you know you like or would like to try. Then look at the meal ideas and corresponding recipes and see which ones appeal to you. The meal ideas and recipes are there to provide inspiration and guidance, but you can create your own meals and recipes as long as you stick with the foods listed and the recommended portion sizes.

Write down exactly what you plan to eat for all your meals and snacks for the first five days. You'll do this again for the second five days of the challenge. Making big diet changes can be physically and emotionally challenging for a lot of people and you may experience physical and emotional withdrawal symptoms, so it's vital that you do everything you can to lessen your workload and stress levels while on the challenge. Planning ahead like this will help.

If you don't plan ahead, you put yourself in the position of having to make choices and solve problems in the moment, and I think you'll agree that when you're tired and hungry, you're a lot less likely to make good food choices.

• Food shopping •

Once you've filled out your meal plan, make a comprehensive shopping list for food items. Initially you may need to make a trip to both the supermarket and the health food store to stock up on the foods and drinks you'll need. Decide *when* and *where* you're going to shop and *make time* in your schedule to do so.

• Utensils and storage •

You don't need any specific cooking equipment or utensils beyond what would normally feature in an ordinary kitchen, though I do recommend that you buy a set of measuring cups to help you gauge portion sizes. If you don't already have one, invest in a steamer for your veggies. You can buy a three-tiered steamer pot very cheaply. They're handy and economical, as you can cook a number of different items at the same time in the one pot. I'd be lost without mine.

If you plan to make smoothies, hummus or guacamole, then a blender is probably necessary. You should also invest in some good storage containers in a range of different sizes so that you can easily transport lunch, snacks, etc. when out and about.

•Freezing and batch cooking •

If, like most people, you are time starved or sometimes feel too tired to cook from scratch in the evenings, then cook a few dinners, soups, etc. in advance and freeze them so you have healthy options to hand at all times.

For example, whenever I make a up a Bolognese sauce or a curry, I cook double the amount and either store it in the fridge to eat a day or so later or else freeze it for later use. This is so handy, especially on days when you know that you're likely to be particularly busy or tired.

•Healthy snacks •

Get into the habit of keeping healthy snacks close to hand at all times so you will have no excuse when hunger and temptation strike. I always carry a container with nuts, oat cakes and fruit in my handbag so that I don't get caught out and tempted to reach for the biscuit tin. You may also like to keep a few healthy snacks in your car or at your work desk too.

• Create time to succeed •

Changing your eating habits goes way beyond just eating differently. In order to succeed, you'll need to dedicate time to plan meals, shop for food and cook. This takes time and energy, which can be challenging, especially in the beginning. Don't assume this time and energy will magically appear and make itself available to you.

If you're like most people, your days are probably already full with work, children, family responsibilities, housework, social events and hobbies. You will need to create some extra time for yourself by taking a good look at your schedule and re-evaluating priorities, at least initially, until you're in the swing of things. Clearing time in your schedule will often mean decreasing or eliminating some activities, delegating tasks and practising smart time management.

If you have trouble figuring out how to clear some extra time in your schedule, making a priority chart can really help. First write down all the tasks and activities you do in a given day or week. Then divide these tasks and activities into two categories: essential and desirable. You may find that many tasks you had always thought of as essential are actually just desirable and you can afford to cut back on them for the next couple of weeks until you've settled into your new way of eating.

For example, take Susan. Susan is 42, works full time and has a seven-year-old daughter, Amy. She often struggles to meet the demands of work and family life and feels her diet and health have suffered as a result. Look at how Susan divided up her daily tasks and activities.

Essential

Work

Mother duties: get Amy dressed and ready for school, drop off and collect from school

Help Amy with her homework

Essential housework: do the dishes, hoovering, mopping, laundry, ironing and make beds

Food shopping

Prepare meals/cooking

Pay household bills

Amy's bedtime routine

Desirable

Check social media (Facebook and Twitter)

Watch TV

Surf the internet

Have a bubble bath

Go to the playground

Organise slumber party for Amy

Drive Amy to and from drama class

Read my book

Visit my mother

Call my friend

Clean out the attic

Paint the front door

Go to the cinema

So how did Susan clear some time in her schedule for her new eating plan? She did some clever problem-solving and delegating. Firstly, she got out of bed 10 minutes earlier on weekdays to give herself time to prepare and pack a healthy lunch to take to work. She didn't particularly like doing this at first, but when it came to lunchtime she was very glad to have her healthy packed lunch with her.

Then Susan decided to do some delegating. She asked her husband to take over Amy's bedtime routine on weeknights, which meant she had an extra 15 minutes every evening to plan meals for the next day and make her food shop list.

Next, Susan spoke with a mum from her daughter's drama group and organised that they would take turns dropping off and collecting the girls. This meant that every second Saturday, Anna had free time to do some batch cooking. This was a saving grace, particularly on Thursday evenings when she worked late and felt too tired to cook.

Susan also recognised that while it would be desirable to clean out the attic and paint the front door at the weekend, it just wasn't a priority right now and could be put on the back burner for another few weeks. Once she made that decision, it took a lot of pressure off and she stopped feeling guilty at weekends for not doing more work around the house.

Susan also thought about all the things she liked to do in the evenings as part of her valuable 'me time'. She recognised that she enjoyed watching a bit of telly in the evenings with her husband and reading before bed helped her to fall asleep. But when she thought about the amount of time she spent surfing the net and on Facebook, she realised that she didn't really get all that much out of doing it and so she decided to use some of the time she'd normally spend online to read her **benefits list** instead. She found this really kept her focused and kept her motivation levels up.

Finally, instead of phoning her best friend once a week and spending an hour on the phone, Susan suggested that they meet up for a walk once a week instead and get an hour's exercise in while catching up. Her friend was happy to oblige and enjoyed the exercise too.

If lack of time is a potential challenge for you, it's worth thinking about how you plan to overcome this. As you can see, Susan only made a few small changes to her schedule, but sometimes you only have to change a little to change a lot. Those small changes could be the difference between success and failure.

'THE KEY IS NOT

TO PRIORITISE WHAT'S

ON YOUR SCHEDULE, BUT TO

SCHEDULE YOUR PRIORITIES.'

STEPHEN COVEY

• Lose the guilt •

Last but not least, if you feel guilty about the idea of asking others for help or making yourself a priority over the coming weeks, don't. Remember, everyone close to you will benefit in the long run when you reach your health goals.

If everyone else around you is worthy of care and attention, then so are you. You not only deserve this time, you *need* it for your own health and well-being. Self-time is not selfish, it's a necessary dimension of self-care.

What are you thinking?

Are you having negative or resistant thoughts about making changes to your schedule or environment? If so, reframe your thoughts into more positive, helpful ones. Here's an example.

Negative, unhelpful thought:

I don't want to make changes to my schedule. I'm busy enough as it is.

Positive, helpful thought:

I am willing to do what it takes to succeed, even if it requires an initial sacrifice. Being slim and healthy is worth it to me.

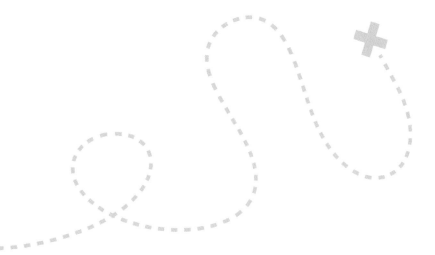

CHAPTER 4

THE 10-DAY SUGAR CHALLENGE

A
LOW-GLYCEMIC
APPROACH

FIVE
GOLDEN
RULES

10-DAY SUGAR
CHALLENGE
FOOD LIST

ADDITIONAL
GUIDELINES

MEAL
SUGGESTIONS

HELPFUL
SUPPLEMENTS

NEXT
STEPS

THE PURPOSE OF the 10-Day Sugar Challenge is to wipe the slate clean and give your body a clear path to restore its own natural balance. Think of it as a fresh start for your body and your mind.

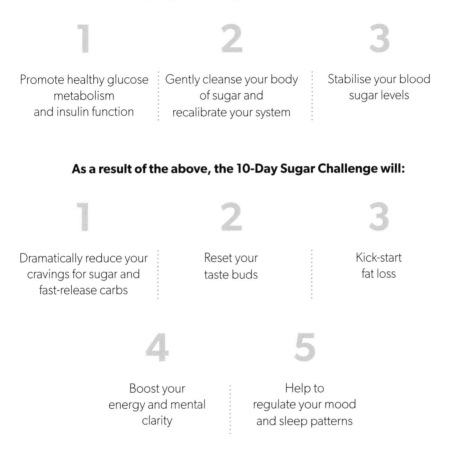

The 10-Day Sugar Challenge has been formulated to:

1 Promote healthy glucose metabolism and insulin function

2 Gently cleanse your body of sugar and recalibrate your system

3 Stabilise your blood sugar levels

As a result of the above, the 10-Day Sugar Challenge will:

1 Dramatically reduce your cravings for sugar and fast-release carbs

2 Reset your taste buds

3 Kick-start fat loss

4 Boost your energy and mental clarity

5 Help to regulate your mood and sleep patterns

To achieve this, it's necessary to eliminate sugar from your diet entirely for a short period of time. The good news is that it only takes 10 days to kick-start this process and my sugar challenge won't leave you hungry or slow down your metabolism. On the contrary, you'll have plenty of tasty and nutritious foods to eat – normal, everyday foods. No shakes, no pills, no off-limits food groups, just a simple, practical and satisfying eating plan that will gently balance your blood sugar and reset your metabolism. By eating the correct balance of quality protein, healthy fats and good carbohydrates, your body simply won't crave sugar or fast-release carbohydrates the way it used to.

A low-glycemic approach

THE 10-DAY SUGAR CHALLENGE is largely made up of low-glycemic foods, which are the best foods to keep blood sugars stable and therefore minimise cravings for sugar. For this reason, low-glycemic foods can be viewed as low-trigger foods, as they are unlikely to trigger any cravings for sugar.

You're probably already familiar with the terms *glycemic index* and *glycemic load*, but these terms often cause confusion. Allow me to explain the difference. In a nutshell, both are numerical systems of measuring the degree to which a carbohydrate is likely to raise your blood sugar and insulin levels. So a low-GI/GL food will cause a small rise in blood sugar, whereas a high-GI/GL food will trigger a dramatic rise (spike) in blood sugar. The idea of both rating systems is to help you choose foods that will keep your blood sugar levels stable.

The main difference is that the glycemic index rates a food as a whole (e.g. an entire watermelon), whereas the glycemic load rates a food based on a typical serving size (e.g. 2 slices of watermelon), which gives you a more accurate and practical picture.

As a general rule of thumb, slow-release carbohydrates (e.g. oats, brown rice and quinoa) will have a low to medium GI/GL score, whereas fast-release carbohydrates (e.g. white bread, white pasta and cornflakes) will have a high GI/GL score.

But you don't need to get bogged down with these rating systems or start counting scores. I've done the work for you. The foods listed on the 10-Day Sugar Challenge and the meal suggestions and recipes I've given you focus on low-glycemic foods that will keep your blood sugars stable and stave off cravings.

Health benefits of a low-glycemic diet

In addition to weight loss, a low-glycemic diet is associated with better blood sugar and insulin control, increased energy, improved mood and disease prevention. In fact, a large review of 37 scientific studies on the effects of the glycemic index and glycemic load on disease prevention showed that following a low-glycemic diet independently reduces a person's risk for type 2 diabetes, coronary heart disease, gallbladder disease and breast cancer.

• Withdrawal symptoms •

You may experience some withdrawal symptoms for a few days, such as headaches, nausea and fatigue, as your system gently detoxifies and rebalances itself. Try to take it easy for those first few days and drink plenty of water. This programme is designed to support your body as it gently cleanses itself, so the withdrawal symptoms won't last long and you won't go hungry.

BY THE END OF IT, YOU'LL
FEEL CLEAN, EMPOWERED AND IN
CONTROL. AND AS A BONUS, IT'S
LIKELY TO KICK-START WEIGHT LOSS
TOO IF YOU'RE CARRYING EXTRA
WEIGHT, WHICH WILL GIVE YOUR
MOTIVATION LEVELS A NICE BOOST.

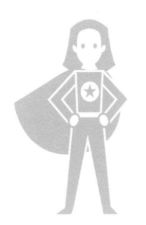

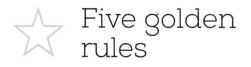 # Five golden rules

To follow the 10-Day Sugar Challenge, all you need to do is follow the five golden rules.

1. Stick to the foods listed on the plan

On pages 48–49 you'll find a list of all the nutritious foods you can eat on the 10-Day Sugar Challenge. You may be wondering if you can eat and drink this or that, so I'll keep this very simple: if it's not on the list, don't eat or drink it. The foods listed are low-glycemic foods designed to help keep your blood sugar and insulin levels stable so as to minimise cravings and keep you full and satisfied. If a food isn't listed, it means that it didn't meet specific criteria in terms of its glycemic rating or its nutritional value. Bread, pasta and potatoes are off limits for 10 days only.

Also, you'll notice that most of the foods listed are unprocessed, natural whole foods. You won't feel the amazing effects of this challenge if you choose to eat highly processed foods. The natural foods on the list will nourish your cells, boost your energy and support your body as it gently detoxifies. There are numerous ways to make this plan work for you and I'll be showing you exactly how to put it all into practice.

2. Include a portion of protein with every meal and snack

As well as being filling, protein helps stabilise blood sugar and thus significantly reduces cravings for starchy and sweet foods. Protein also provides the building blocks for brain chemicals that influence appetite and satiety. The 'Additional guidelines' section on pages 50–55 will tell you the types of protein you should eat and how much.

3. Get the balance right at mealtimes

In order to have a balanced diet, you need to ensure that each of your meals is nutritionally balanced. A nutritionally balanced meal is one that contains the correct balance (i.e. proportions) of protein, carbohydrates and fat and includes plenty of vegetables for added fibre and nutrition. Eating the proper ratio of protein, carbohydrates and fats at mealtimes keeps blood sugar stable, stops food cravings and sustains energy levels.

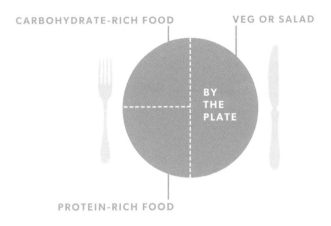

Here's how to divide your plate for a balanced meal:

- One-quarter of your meal should consist of **protein-rich food(s)** such as fish, eggs, meat, tofu or a serving of beans or lentils. You can combine various proteins if you wish.
- Another quarter of your meal should contain **slow-release carbohydrates**, such as brown rice, quinoa, bulgur wheat, oats or pearl barley. (See the food list on page 48 for carbohydrate options.)
- The remaining half of your meal should be made up of vegetables, ideally non-starchy vegetables as listed on the food list on page 49.

The 'Additional guidelines' section will explain how you can incorporate moderate amounts of healthy fats into your meals and snacks.

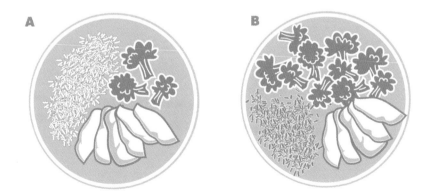

Does your plate look more like A or B? You should aim to model your plate after B.

4. Eat every two to three hours

An essential part of keeping your blood sugar levels stable and staving off hunger and cravings is to eat approximately every two to three hours. Three main meals per day and two snacks is ideal. This will keep your metabolism and energy levels up. The sample menu on the next page illustrates how to put this into practice.

TOP TIP:

ALWAYS HAVE HEALTHY SNACKS

CLOSE TO HAND SO THAT YOU HAVE

NO EXCUSE WHEN TEMPTATION

STRIKES! HEALTHY SNACK OPTIONS

ARE LISTED ON PAGE 58.

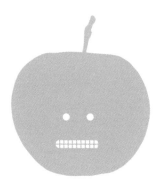

Breakfast – 8.00am
Bowl of porridge topped with berries and milled seeds

Mid-morning snack – 11.00am
A palmful of almonds and an apple

Lunch – 1.00pm
Chicken, vegetable and barley soup

Mid-afternoon snack – 4.00pm
Hummus on oat crackers

Dinner – 7.00pm
Beef and veggie stir-fry with brown rice

5. Limit stimulants and alcohol

Sugar isn't the only thing that can upset your blood sugar levels. Stimulants such as caffeine and nicotine increase levels of the stress hormones adrenalin and cortisol, which can interfere with your blood sugar balance and wreak havoc on your nervous system, thereby making you more prone to stress and anxiety.

When it comes to caffeinated drinks such as tea and coffee, it would be best to cut them out altogether to get the most out of the 10-Day Sugar Challenge. But if it feels like it would be too much for you to eliminate caffeine entirely, then try to cut your consumption down to no more than two cups a day of either tea or coffee, ideally less.

A good way to gently wean yourself off caffeine and minimise withdrawal symptoms is to alternate every second cup of tea or coffee with a caffeine-free herbal tea instead. Another option is to reduce the number of espresso shots in your coffee to a single shot only. And of course, don't add sugar or sweeteners to your tea or coffee.

All soft drinks, sodas, energy drinks, cordials and juices, including diet versions, are strictly off limits.

You should also avoid all alcohol for the duration of the 10-Day Sugar Challenge. Alcohol upsets blood sugar balance, increases appetite and weakens resolve. It can be reintroduced afterwards in moderation. I cover alcohol in more detail in Chapter 6.

10-Day Sugar Challenge food list

BY NOW, I bet you're dying to know what you can eat on the 10-Day Sugar Challenge. Here is a list of foods for you to choose from.

Meat, poultry and eggs

Beef	Chicken
Pork	Turkey
Lamb	Pheasant
Duck	Goose
Venison	Quail
Bacon*	Eggs (chicken, duck,
Ham*	goose, quail)
Veal	

See the additional guidelines on page 51 for recommendations regarding processed meats.

Fish

All types of fresh fish are allowed, including but not limited to:

Salmon	Cod
Prawns	Scallops
Tuna	Swordfish
Halibut	Monkfish
Hake	Seabass
Sardines	Kippers
Whiting	Oysters
Mussels	Trout
Sole	Haddock
Crab	Lobster

See the additional guidelines on page 52 for recommendations on fish.

Carbohydrate-rich food (slow-releasing)

Brown rice, oats, quinoa, pearl barley, bulgur wheat, amaranth, millet, oatcakes, rye crispbread (sugar-free)

Beans, lentils, soy products

Beans: Kidney, black, red, navy, pinto, cannellini, soy, butter, chickpeas
Lentils: Brown, green, red, yellow
Soy products: Tofu, tempeh

See the additional guidelines on page 52 for portion control and cooking methods.

Nuts, seeds and butters

Nuts: Walnut, almond, chestnut, brazil, peanut, pecan, hazelnut, macadamia, pine, pistachio, cashew
Seeds: Flax, chia, sesame, sunflower, pumpkin, hemp, poppy
Nut/seed butters: Butters made from the nuts and seeds above are allowed, e.g. almond butter, peanut butter, tahini

See the additional guidelines on page 52 for recommended portions.

Fruit

Strawberry	Raspberry
Blueberry	Blackberry
Lemon and lime	Green apple
Grapefruit	Avocado
Plum	

See the additional guidelines on page 53 for further recommendations on fruit.

Fats and oils

Olive, rapeseed, sesame, coconut, flax and hemp oils (preferably cold-pressed)

Vegetables

Peppers	Courgettes
Green beans	Asparagus
Broccoli	Artichokes
Onions	Brussels sprouts
Scallions	Chilli peppers
Tomatoes	Cabbage
Cauliflower	Celery
Aubergines	Leeks
Garlic	Lettuce
Green salads	Kale
Ginger	Spinach
Snap peas	Mangetout
Mushrooms	Lemongrass
Chillis	Capers
Carrots*	Alfalfa sprouts
Bok choy	Chives
Cucumbers	Fennel
Radishes	Bamboo shoots
Chard	Okra
Olives	Sauerkraut
	(raw and sugar-free)

See the additional guidelines on page 53 for further recommendations on carrots.

Dairy

Cow's milk, all cow's milk cheese, butter, natural unsweetened yoghurt or kefir, goat's milk, all goat's milk cheese, sheep's milk, all sheep's milk cheese, buffalo milk, mozzarella

See the additional guidelines on page 54 for further advice and portion guidelines.

Dairy alternatives

Non-dairy milks: Soy, oat, almond, coconut, hemp, hazelnut, cashew, quinoa (choose unsweetened varieties)

Herbs, spices, stocks and vinegars

All natural herbs and spices
  (fresh or dried)
Preservative-free, low-salt stock
  or bouillon
Naturally brewed soy sauce or tamari
Dijon or plain mustard (choose sugar-
  or honey-free varieties)
Mayonnaise (choose full-fat, sugar-free
  varieties and limit to 1 teaspoon
  per day)
Vinegars: White, cider, wine,
  balsamic (limit balsamic vinegar to
  1 tablespoon per day)

Beverages

Tea, coffee or green tea: 2 caffeinated
  drinks per day at most
Herbal teas (choose sugar- and
  caffeine-free varieties)
Filtered water
Sparkling water

See the additional guidelines on page 55 for extra notes on beverages.

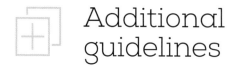

Additional guidelines

• Protein portion guidelines •

A simple way to gauge how much protein you should eat at mealtimes involves your hand. In a nutshell, the portion of protein you should aim to eat at lunch and dinner should be roughly the size of the palm of your hand. The divided plate shown in Figure B on page 45 is another way of helping you gauge portion size and amounts.

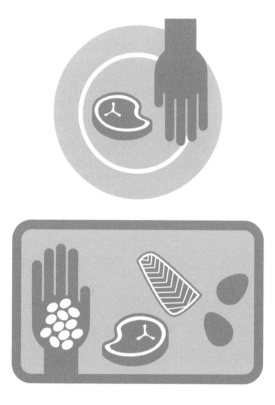

Consuming a palm-sized portion of protein at breakfast isn't always practical or even necessary. The breakfast suggestions and recipes I've given you all contain adequate amounts of protein to ensure you'll be eating a balanced breakfast.

Similarly, all of the snack suggestions incorporate just enough protein (about half a palm-sized portion) to help keep your blood sugar stable and reduce hunger and cravings.

• Animal vs. plant protein •

The main sources of animal and plant protein are:
• **Animal protein:** Meat, fish, poultry, eggs, dairy
• **Plant protein:** Beans, lentils, nuts, seeds, tofu, tempeh
From a general health perspective, you should strive for a relatively even balance between animal sources of protein and plant sources of protein (unless you are a vegetarian or vegan, of course). Consuming too much animal protein isn't good for your health, so you should eat plant sources of protein too. Plant sources of protein like beans, lentils, nuts and seeds are associated with increased health and longevity because they are loaded with vitamins, minerals and fibre and as such should form a valuable part of a healthy and balanced diet.

Personally, I strive for a 50–50 balance between animal and plant protein in my diet. Play around and see what balance works best for you. If you're not used to eating plant sources of protein, fear not, as you will find simple and delicious ways to incorporate these foods into your diet with the meal suggestions and recipes I'll be giving you. The sample menu on page 47 is a good example of a diet that contains healthy amounts of both animal and plant protein.

• Meat: Quantity and quality •

Where meat and poultry are concerned, always choose lean cuts and trim excess fat. I recommend no more than two servings of red meat per week.

• Processed meats •

If you choose to eat processed versions of the meats listed on the plan, such as cured or smoked bacon, ham or chicken, you should only do so in very strict moderation, as processed meats tend to be high in salt and preservatives. Avoid those cured with sugar and steer clear of meats with added nitrates.

•Eggs •

Current research indicates that up to seven eggs per week can be eaten as part of a healthy and balanced diet.

• Fish •

Fresh fish is always best if possible. Frozen fish is fine provided the fish is not crumbed or coated. Tinned fish is also acceptable, but ideally choose varieties tinned in water. If it's tinned in brine or oil, drain off the excess before eating.

Fish that is cured, smoked or pickled is typically high in sodium and should be consumed in moderation, particularly for those with high blood pressure.

Oily fish such as salmon, mackerel, trout and sardines are high in omega-3 fats, which are known to boost mood and concentration as well as improve cardiovascular health. For this reason, I recommend that you consume two portions of oily fish per week for optimal nutrition and health. If you don't eat fish, you should take a good-quality omega-3 fish oil supplement.

• Beans and lentils •

Beans and lentils are unique in that they provide both protein and carbohydrate. However, because of their high fibre content, they are still a relatively low-glycemic food.

½ cup* cooked beans or lentils = 1 portion

Try to limit your consumption to one portion per day on the 10-Day Sugar Challenge. However, vegetarians may wish to have two portions per day, which is acceptable.

Dried beans and lentils (ideally soaked overnight) are preferable to canned varieties, as there will be less of an impact on blood sugar and the benefits to gut flora will be maximised. Soaking also removes some of the substances that cause flatulence and assists in nutrient absorption. That said, canned beans and lentils are still a good option if you're pressed for time. Always choose sugar-free brands and rinse well before use.

Sprouted beans and lentils are also an extremely nutritious and healthful option.

*Always use standard measuring cups, not ordinary teacups or mugs.

• Nuts and seeds •

1 palmful of nuts or seeds = 1 portion
1 tablespoon nut or seed butter = 1 portion

I encourage you to have 1 heaped tablespoon of seeds per day, particularly those high in omega-3 fats, such as chia, flax or hemp seed.

I recommend no more than two portions of nuts and seeds or their butters per day.

Nuts and seeds should be eaten in their natural raw state, i.e. not salted or coated in anything. Where nut and seed butters are concerned, opt for brands with no added salt or sugar.

• Vegetables •

The vegetables listed on the 10-Day Sugar Challenge are predominantly non-starchy, low-glycemic vegetables. As an absolute minimum, you will need to eat at least three portions of vegetables per day. However, for optimal health and disease prevention, you should aim for five portions of vegetables per day.

Don't worry if this is more than what you're used to. You'll discover just how easy it is to incorporate vegetables into your meals and snacks when you follow the meal ideas and recipes.

So what constitutes a portion of vegetables? There are a number of ways to gauge portion size:

½ cup or 3 heaped tablespoons of chopped vegetables (cooked or raw) = 1 portion
1 cup raw leafy vegetables (e.g. spinach, rocket) = 1 portion

Vegetables may be fresh or frozen, but avoid tinned vegetables.

Carrot should be limited to no more than one portion per day, as it is relatively high in naturally occurring sugars and starch. Raw carrot is preferable over cooked carrot in this regard.

• Fruit •

There are temporary restrictions on fruit for the duration of the 10-Day Sugar Challenge because certain fruits are high in natural sugars, which can affect your blood sugar balance and hence trigger cravings. All the fruits listed on the 10-Day Sugar Challenge are low-glycemic fruits that won't spike your blood sugar and will help reset your taste buds away from sweet foods.

Aim for two portions of fruit per day.

1 cup berries = 1 portion
2 plums = 1 portion
½ grapefruit = 1 portion
½ avocado = 1 portion

Avocado doesn't count as part of your daily fruit allowance. Up to four portions of avocado a week may be consumed on top of your fruit allowance. This amounts to two avocados per week. Avocados are high in essential fats and are exceptionally filling and satisfying.

Fruit may be fresh or frozen, but not canned. Strictly avoid all types of dried fruit, fruit juices, squashes and cordials.

• Dairy •

It's not essential to consume dairy on this programme. If you choose to do so, limit your intake to no more than two portions per day.

240ml (8fl oz) milk = 1 portion
125g yoghurt or cottage cheese = 1 portion
½ cup ricotta, feta or goat's cheese = 1 portion
30g Cheddar cheese = 1 portion

Try to choose whole versions of milk and yoghurt over low-fat. Organic is preferable if it's within your budget. Choose natural yoghurts with no added sugar and preferably probiotic ones to boost digestive health.

I favour natural, full-fat butter over low-fat spreads in terms of its nutritional value and the quality of the fat. Limit butter to a maximum of one pat or 1 teaspoon per day (1 teaspoon of butter can be consumed on top of your two portions of dairy).

• Slow-release carbohydrates portion guide •

I recommend consuming between two and four portions of the slow-release carbohydrates listed on the plan per day, depending on your activity level and/or whether or not you need to lose weight. Use a measuring cup in the early stages.

½ cup oats (approx. 40g) = 1 portion
½ cup (approx. 3 heaped tablespoons) cooked rice, quinoa,
   barley or bulgur wheat = 1 portion
2 oat or rye crackers = ½ portion (e.g. as a snack or a side)
4 oat or rye crackers = 1 portion

ENERGY MODIFICATIONS BASED ON ACTIVITY LEVEL

If you have a very active lifestyle, work at a physically demanding job and/or regularly participate in high-intensity physical activity or exercise, you will probably need to consume four portions of carbohydrate-rich food per day. Also, in terms of dividing your plate, your portion of carbohydrate-rich food may take up a little more than one-quarter of the plate, such as two-thirds of a cup of rice.

Please note that these guidelines are estimates only. If you find that you need more carbohydrates to maintain your activity level, adjust according to your needs.

Here is a sample menu that includes four portions of carbohydrate-rich food (in red):

Breakfast: Porridge **oats** with berries and mixed seeds
Snack: 2 **oatcakes** with peanut butter and sliced apple
Lunch: Chicken, vegetable and **barley** soup (page 157)
Snack: 2 **oatcakes** with cheese or hummus
Dinner: Red lentil curry with **brown rice** (page 168)

WEIGHT LOSS MODIFICATIONS

If you need to lose weight, limit yourself to two or three portions of carbohydrate-rich foods per day until you reach your goal weight. This may mean omitting a portion of carbohydrate-rich food from one meal per day and substituting it with more vegetables or beans or lentils instead.

Here is a sample menu that includes two portions of carbohydrate-rich food (in red):

Breakfast: Natural yoghurt topped with sugar-free granola and fruit (page 148)

Snack: Palmful of cashew nuts and 2 plums

Lunch: Tuna salad

Snack: Hummus (page 187) and celery sticks

Dinner: Cheesy chicken and veggie bake (page 174)

• Fats and oils •

Limit your consumption of the oils listed on the plan to between 1 and 2 tablespoons per day. Olive or coconut oil are the best options. Along with regularly consuming modest portions of seeds, nuts, oily fish and avocado, this will ensure that you are consuming the right amount of fat (including essential fatty acids) for a balanced diet and optimum nutrition.

• Beverages •

Aim to drink between 1.5 to 2 litres of pure filtered water per day. Herbal teas count as part of this. Sparkling water is allowed.

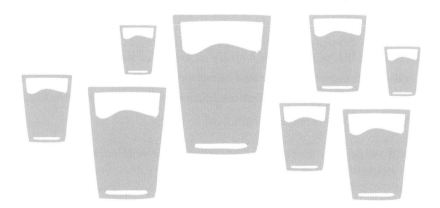

Meal suggestions

THE FOLLOWING ARE suggested meal and snack options for the 10-Day Sugar Challenge. These suggestions are meant as ideas only. Feel free to use the guidelines and come up with your own creations.

• Breakfast •

- **Porridge oats + milk of choice, cinnamon, grated apple and 1 tablespoon milled seeds**
- **Supercharger smoothie (page 152)**
- **Milk or yoghurt topped with sugar-free granola and berries (page 148)**
- **Boiled or scrambled egg with grilled tomato or mushroom served with 2 oatcakes**
- **1 power pancake (page 151)**
- **3 oatcakes topped with cheese and an apple**
- **Scrambled egg with smoked salmon and avocado**
- **3 oatcakes topped with peanut butter and apple**

• Lunch •

SALADS

1. **Choose a portion of protein.** You can combine a couple of these together. Here are some examples extracted from the main food list on pages 48–49: chicken, turkey, ham, hard-boiled egg, hummus, mozzarella, feta, tuna, salmon, sardines, chickpeas, butter beans, kidney, cannellini beans.
2. **Combine the protein with a range of salads or veggies.** Here are some examples extracted from the main food list: lettuce, mixed leaves, rocket, baby spinach, avocado, tomatoes, peppers, cucumber, onion, grated carrot or courgette, celery, sprouts.
3. **Add a healthy dressing (optional).** See page 190 for simple dressing options.
4. **Add one portion of a carbohydrate-rich food (slow-releasing) to serve with or alongside your salad (optional).** Here are some examples extracted from the main food list: oatcakes, rye crispbread, quinoa, bulgar wheat, brown rice.

SOUPS

Soup is a comforting lunch option, particularly on cold winter days, and it's a great way to get your veggies in and meet your five a day. Just make sure to always include a source of protein, either within your soup or alongside it, so that it's a balanced meal. The soups in the recipe section will help you do this. In fact, all of the soups listed are complete meals and do not necessarily require sides. For convenience, consider making up a large batch of soup in advance, which you can store in the fridge or freezer. Put some soup into a thermos flask for work or a transportable container that you can reheat in work.

EGGS

Eggs are a great lunch option because they're so versatile, quick to make and filling. Omelettes are particularly flexible. You can eat them plain or with anything from one to a dozen ingredients, including onion, mushroom, tomato, cheese, spinach, herbs, courgette, etc. See my recipe on page 164.

LEFTOVERS

I'm a big fan of making lunch out of leftovers from the night before. I often take this into consideration at dinnertime by cooking a little extra. Or if I fancy a second helping at dinner, I console myself by deciding to have that second helping for lunch instead the following day. That way I get two meals out of what I've cooked and never feel too full.

At the start of the week I often boil up a big pot of quinoa and store it in the fridge so that I can add it to soups and salads at lunchtime and make burgers or bakes out of it for dinner – see the recipe section for ideas. It's also handy to keep a few hard-boiled eggs in the fridge for a speedy meal or snack option.

LUNCH IDEAS

- **Mediterranean white bean and vegetable soup (page 158)**
- **Oatcakes or rye crispbreads topped with hummus (page 187), cheese or tuna with slices of tomato and cucumber on top**
- **Tomato, mozzarella and chickpea salad (page 161)**
- **Chicken, vegetable and barley soup with a hint of ginger (page 157)**
- **Ham, coleslaw and hard-boiled egg salad**
- **Mushroom omelette with cherry tomatoes**
- **Chickpea, quinoa and avocado salad**
- **Bulgur salad with feta and blueberries (page 162)**

• Snack ideas •

- **Natural yoghurt topped with stewed apple and cinnamon or fresh berries**
- **A palmful of nuts or seeds with a green apple or plum**
- **Almond butter spread on sliced green apples**
- **Supercharger smoothie (page 152)**
- **Oatcakes or rye crispbread topped with either hard-boiled egg, cheese, hummus (page 187), nut butter or guacamole (page 189)**
- **Veggie sticks with hummus (page 187) or guacamole (page 189)**

•Dinner •

The two most important things to remember when it comes to dinner is to use fresh, natural ingredients from the 10-Day Sugar Challenge food list and to make sure it's a balanced meal in terms of the amount of protein and carbohydrates it contains. This means filling one-quarter of your dinner plate with protein-rich food, another quarter with carbohydrate-rich food and the remaining half with non-starchy vegetables.

You can keep meals simple or be as adventurous as you like. Here are some suggestions, but feel free to come up with your own meal ideas.

DINNER SUGGESTIONS

- **Pork stir-fry with ginger, garlic, onions, peppers, mushrooms and mangetout. Use a dash of soy sauce or tamari and serve with wholegrain basmati rice.**
- **Prosciutto-wrapped cod with warm asparagus salad (page 173)**
- **Lean steak served with fried mushrooms and onions and simple cauliflower mash (page 186)**
- **Red lentil curry (page 168) served with wholegrain basmati rice**
- **Cheesy chicken and veggie bake (page 174)**
- **Healthy shepherd's pie (page 178)**
- **Mediterranean chicken with roasted vegetables (page 180)**
- **Speedy salmon supper (page 181)**
- **Chickpea and quinoa burgers (page 170) served with rocket and cherry tomato salad**
- **Scrumptious veggie omelette (page 164)**

Helpful supplements

AS YOU EMBARK on the 10-Day Sugar Challenge, you may be wondering if there are any supplements that may help with cravings and/or withdrawal symptoms.

I never use, encourage or prescribe any form of diet pills or aids to my clients or readers. I tend to favour gentle and natural functional foods and supplements and always take a 'less is more' approach. Below are a few safe and effective options that my clients have found useful and which are known to support healthy blood sugar metabolism. Please note that it is not essential to use any of these foods or supplements. They are simply options for additional support.

• Cinnamon •

Research has shown that this warm, sweet spice helps to reduce sugar cravings by increasing insulin sensitivity and thus supporting healthy glucose metabolism.

Ceylon cinnamon, which you can buy in health food stores or online, is the true form of cinnamon and the one I recommend you use. Cassia cinnamon is the type you'll find in most supermarkets. Cassia cinnamon can contain fairly substantial amounts of a chemical called coumarin. In people who are sensitive, coumarin may cause or worsen liver disease if consumed in large amounts, so it's best to stick with Ceylon cinnamon, particularly if you're consuming a fair amount of it on a regular basis.

Naturally sweet and delightfully aromatic, cinnamon adds beautiful flavour and a hint of sweetness to a variety of food. It works particularly well sprinkled over porridge, yoghurt, smoothies, hot milk and also in curries and marinades. Add 1–2 teaspoons per day to whichever foods or drinks you like.

You can also make or buy cinnamon tea, which I personally find comforting for the way it tastes and also for its wonderful aroma.

• Chromium •

Chromium is a mineral that helps you maintain blood sugar control and staves off sugar cravings. Chromium is found naturally in foods such as beans, nuts, seeds, eggs, onions, asparagus and mushrooms.

However, you can help maintain blood sugar control and reduce sweet cravings more quickly and effectively by taking it in supplement form. The best form of supplementary chromium is chromium picolinate. I recommend taking one 200mcg capsule twice a day for the first month or two to help support your dietary changes, particularly if you are struggling with sugar cravings. It's best taken along with your mid-morning and mid-afternoon snack.

• Magnesium •

Another mineral that is essential for supporting healthy blood sugar metabolism is magnesium. In a nutshell, blood sugar management is much easier when you have enough magnesium in your body. However, many people are deficient in magnesium, particularly those with high-sugar diets and/or high stress levels. This is because high sugar and stress levels in the body increase the excretion of magnesium by the kidneys.

Good dietary sources of magnesium include spinach, broccoli, Swiss chard, sunflower seeds and pumpkin seeds.

As a supplement, I recommend taking between 200mg and 400mg of magnesium citrate per day. Magnesium can be taken at any time of the day, but because of its relaxing effect, I generally recommend taking it in the evening around 30 to 60 minutes before you go to bed.

•

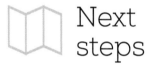

Next steps

SO NOW YOU know exactly what you need to do in order to follow the 10-Day Sugar Challenge. I hope you're feeling excited! If you're feeling a bit daunted, that's perfectly natural too. You may be worrying about how you're going to handle things like cravings and comfort eating – the very things that have probably held you back in the past. Don't worry, though, because I've got you covered.

The next chapter is designed to help solve the problems that have made 'dieting' difficult for you in the past. You'll learn how to overcome emotional eating and resist cravings with ease. The mental skills you'll learn in the next chapter will be critical to your long-term success and will help you succeed where other 'diets' have failed.

What are you thinking?

It's normal to feel daunted or overwhelmed at the thought of making changes to your diet and lifestyle, but don't let these thoughts hold you back from achieving your goals. Try reframing any sabotaging thoughts that pop into your head. Here's an example.

Negative, unhelpful thought:

I don't think I'll be able to do this. It's just too hard.

Positive, helpful thought:

I'm just feeling overwhelmed right now. Yes, this is going to take some getting used to, but once I start seeing and feeling the benefits, it will get easier. What have I got to lose by giving it a go?

CHAPTER 5

CONQUER EMOTIONAL EATING FOR GOOD

EMOTIONAL
VS. PHYSICAL
HUNGER

COMMON
CAUSES OF
EMOTIONAL
EATING

HOW TO
IDENTIFY
YOUR OWN
PERSONAL
TRIGGERS

HOW TO
MANAGE
YOUR
EMOTIONS
WITHOUT
FOOD

HOW TO
RESIST
CRAVINGS

Emotional vs. physical hunger

IF YOU'RE LIKE most people who struggle with a sugar habit, a lot of your eating behaviour is probably driven by emotional hunger as opposed to physical hunger. In other words, you don't choose to eat sugary foods just because you're physically hungry. You choose to eat sugary foods because you want to change or enhance the way you feel.

To overcome emotional eating, you first need to learn how to distinguish between emotional and physical hunger. This can be harder than it sounds, especially if you regularly use food to deal with your feelings. As soon as you're able to recognise whether you are experiencing true hunger vs. emotional hunger, you'll be in a better position to manage your responses accordingly. If you have trouble differentiating between them, don't worry. It just takes a little practice and will become automatic for you in time.

Emotional hunger can be powerful, so it's easy to mistake it for physical hunger. But there are clues you can look for that can help you tell them apart. The table on the next page is a great tool when trying to determine if your hunger is stemming from a physical need to eat or an emotional need to eat.

For the next while, check in with yourself each time you feel like you want to eat something and ask yourself whether you are experiencing physical or emotional hunger.

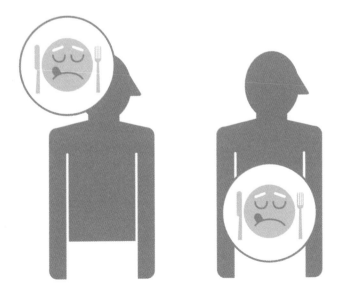

Emotional hunger	Physical hunger
Emotional hunger comes on **suddenly**.	Physical hunger comes on **gradually**. Your stomach starts to feel a little empty, then one hour later it starts to growl. You have progressive clues that you are hungry.
Emotional hunger involves cravings for **specific** comfort foods, e.g. chocolate, ice cream, crisps.	Physical hunger is **flexible**. You may have preferences for what you'd like to eat, but you're open to options.
Emotional hunger is **urgent** and feels like it needs to be satisfied instantly.	Physical hunger is **patient**. You'd rather eat soon, but you don't need to eat right at that very instant.
Emotional hunger starts in the **mouth** and **mind**. Your mouth wants to taste the food and you can't get it off your mind.	Physical hunger starts with **stomach** sensations, i.e. you feel emptiness, gnawing and rumbling sensations.
Emotional hunger arises from an **emotional need**. It can be a positive emotion, e.g. relief, but it's often a negative or uncomfortable one, e.g. stress, boredom, frustration, tiredness, dissatisfaction, emptiness, anger, loneliness, shame.	Physical hunger arises out of a **physical need** resulting from a low level of glucose in the bloodstream.
Emotional hunger often involves **mindless** or **automatic eating**. You may not even realise you've eaten an entire packet of biscuits until they're gone.	Physical hunger involves **deliberate choices** and an **awareness** of the food you are eating and how much of it you eat.
Emotional hunger **doesn't stop even when you're full**. It usually requires you to overeat in order to feel satisfied.	Physical hunger **stops when you're full**.
Emotional hunger **usually involves regret** after you've eaten and often triggers feelings of guilt, powerlessness and shame.	Physical hunger **doesn't involve regret or guilt** because eating to satisfy physical hunger doesn't make you feel bad about yourself.

So where do you start if you want to stop eating emotionally? It may sound like a cliché, but the first step really is awareness – in other words, simply recognising that you do eat emotionally and to what extent.

The next step is identifying your own **personal triggers** because we all eat for a variety of different reasons that are unique to us. For example, some people overeat when stressed whereas others will under-eat. You may really enjoy eating in the company of others or perhaps you prefer eating alone.

Take a moment to think about what feelings make you reach for comfort food. Are there certain situations, people or places that trigger these feelings?

Bear in mind that while most emotional eating is linked to uncomfortable or unpleasant feelings, it can also be triggered by positive emotions such as rewarding yourself for completing a difficult task or a holiday or celebration.

Below is a list of common triggers of emotional eating. See which ones you can relate to.

•

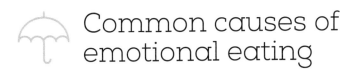

Common causes of emotional eating

• Stress •

Many of us use food as a way to cope with the stresses of everyday life. You start the day with great intentions, but then real-life challenges get in the way and your good intentions go out the window. For example, you planned to have porridge for breakfast but then you get stuck in rush hour traffic and decide to comfort yourself with a muffin when you arrive at work. Or you mindlessly munch through a packet of biscuits to help deal with the pressure of a mounting deadline or tuck into some chocolate after putting a difficult child to bed. It's the classic 'I was doing fine until X happened'. The more unmanaged stress you have in your life, the more likely you are to turn to food for emotional relief.

• Filling a void •

Do you ever eat simply to give yourself something to do or as a way to fill a void in your life? You may feel unfulfilled, bored or dissatisfied with certain aspects of your life and food is an easy way to occupy your mouth and your time. You may feel as though something is missing, but you don't know what that something is. In the moment, food fills up that empty feeling and distracts you from underlying feelings of dissatisfaction. It's an easily found and guaranteed source of pleasure. Perhaps it's the *main* source of pleasure in your life right now.

• Social influences •

Certain people, places or events can trigger you to emotional eat. For example, you're at a party and get so excited by the selection of yummy foods on the buffet table that you get on a high, lose the run of yourself and end up overeating because you want to keep that good feeling going. Or you automatically feel driven to eat every time you go to the cinema because everyone around you seems to be indulging in ice cream and popcorn and you don't want to feel deprived. Perhaps you associate watching a movie with having treats and feel you wouldn't be able to enjoy the movie without the food or you simply want to enhance the experience.

You may also overeat in social situations out of nervousness or social anxiety. Or perhaps your family or circle of friends encourage you to eat a certain way and it's just easier to go along with the group.

• Childhood habits •

Childhood eating habits often carry over into adulthood, particularly eating habits that are charged with emotion. Think back to your childhood memories of food. Were you given sweets if you were feeling sad or rewarded with pizza or ice cream if you did something good? A child who is given a sweet treat after an achievement may grow up using the same types of food as a reward for getting through or achieving something.

Or perhaps you were denied the foods you wanted as a child and felt deprived, and now as an adult you over-eat those foods to compensate or to rebel against food restrictions from your childhood.

Emotional eating can be driven by nostalgia too. For example, you may want to recapture the feeling of baking fairy cakes with your mother or eating ice cream cones at the beach as a child.

How to identify your own personal triggers

YOU PROBABLY RELATED to one or more of the triggers listed above, but you'll need to get more specific in identifying your own personal triggers in order to overcome them. One of the best ways to identify the patterns behind your emotional eating is to keep track with a Food & Mood Journal. All you need is a notebook and pen to create your own.

Every time you eat unhealthy foods, overeat or feel an urge to reach for comfort food, pause for a moment and think back to what may have triggered the urge. If you backtrack a little, you should be able to identify a specific event and/or thought that kicked off the emotional eating cycle. Write it all down in your own Food & Mood Journal. It's best to include the date and time, what you ate or wanted to eat, how you felt beforehand, what you felt as you were eating and how you felt afterwards.

The purpose of keeping a journal is that over time, you'll begin to see patterns emerge. It could be certain times of the day, days of the week, certain people, situations, events, etc. that trigger negative or sabotaging thoughts in you. It could be one type of thought that comes up time and time again or a variety of different thoughts that are holding you back. Keeping a journal will help you identify the real root cause(s) of your emotional eating. Once you know, you'll be in a much stronger position to overcome them.

Below are examples of Food & Mood Journals that Susan and Sean kept while following my programme. This journal template is to guide you, but feel free to create yours any way you want.

Susan's Food & Mood Journal

Date and time	Place and relevant people	Food or beverage craving	Thoughts beforehand	Feelings beforehand	External events that triggered thoughts or feeling	Did I eat? If so, how much? If not, how did I overcome it?	How did I feel afterwards?
20 October 4pm	Having tea in my mother's house	Chocolate digestives	Does she think I'm a bad mother? Am I a bad mother? Why does she always criticise me?	Annoyance, anger, hurt	My mother commenting that my daughter spends too much time watching TV and should be doing more sports	Yes, I ate 4 biscuits with my tea	Really annoyed and frustrated with myself
9pm	At home on the couch after I put Amy to bed	Chocolate	Why does it have to be such a battle getting her to bed? Why can't I get her to bed at a normal hour like other parents? Am I doing something wrong? Why does my husband always leave the bedtime routine to me? It's not fair.	Weary, frustrated, feel like a failure, resentful	My daughter refusing to go to bed, the length of time it took to do bedtime routine and get her to sleep	No, I didn't eat. I read my benefits list, which reminded me of all the positive things I gain by eating healthily. I had a bubble bath instead.	Really proud of myself for not giving in. Relaxed after the bath.

My day in review

What external factors influenced my eating today?
Visiting my mother.

What thoughts and feelings arose as a result?
I mainly thought 'Does she think I'm a bad mother?', then feelings of anger, annoyance and hurt.

What can I learn from today? For example, are there issues that need to be looked at further? Is there anything I could do differently?
Today I learned that I turn to sweet foods when I'm annoyed or upset. I also learned that eating them doesn't make me feel better for more than a few minutes. In fact, it made me feel worse afterwards because then I had two problems: the fact that I was upset and the fact that I'd just eaten something I knew I shouldn't have.

I also learned how good it made me feel NOT to give in to my chocolate craving this evening. Reading my benefits list helped. I realised that there are other ways to make myself feel better besides chocolate, which sounds obvious but was a bit of a revelation for me. I think I need to give some thought as to *why* my mother's comment today upset me so much. Is it because she might have a point about Amy watching too much TV? Maybe this is a separate issue I need to give some thought to.

Sean's Food & Mood Journal

Date and time	Place and relevant people	Food or beverage craving	Thoughts beforehand	Feelings beforehand	External events that triggered thoughts or feeling	Did I eat? If so, how much? If not, how did I overcome it?	How did I feel afterwards?
2 Dec 8.45am	Stuck in traffic jam on way to work	Coffee and croissant	I should have eaten breakfast. I can't stand this traffic. I need to perform well at a presentation this afternoon. I hope I don't get nervous and mess up.	Pressurised, stressed, agitated	Left house without breakfast, stuck in traffic jam, presentation scheduled for the afternoon	Yes, I picked up a coffee and croissant in the café next to the office.	Comforted while I ate, but the coffee made me feel jittery and I felt bloated and stodgy after the croissant.
3.30pm	In office after presentation	Tea and biscuits	I deserve some tea and biscuits after that. I need the sugar and caffeine hit to get me through the rest of the afternoon.	Pleased and relieved I performed well at presentation. Tired.	Finished my presentation, have other work to complete afterwards.	I decided to delay having the tea and biscuits and went for a 5-minute brisk walk around the office grounds instead. When I got back I ate some nuts and fruit.	I felt refreshed and more awake after the walk and didn't crave the tea and biscuits as much. I felt really good about eating the healthy snack and it kept me going till dinner.

My day in review

What external factors influenced my eating today?
Leaving the house without breakfast, getting stuck in traffic and having to give a presentation at work.

What thoughts and feelings arose as a result?
'I can't stand this traffic', 'I need a coffee and a croissant', 'I can't be late', then stress, frustration and pressure.

What can I learn from today? For example, are there issues that need to be looked at further? Is there anything I could do differently?
I need to start getting up earlier to allow time to have breakfast at home so I'm less tempted to get a coffee and pastry at work. I might try leaving the house a little earlier too so I can avoid traffic where possible. Also, maybe I could start viewing the times I do get stuck in traffic a little more positively and use the time to catch up on the news or listen to that self-help audio book that's in my glove compartment.

Not giving in to my craving immediately and distracting myself with a quick walk worked for me today. I didn't want the tea and biscuits half as much after my walk, so I'll try that approach next time I have a craving. Also, having the healthy snacks in my desk drawer made it easier to make the healthy choice.

How to manage your emotions without food

As you begin to get a better understanding of what *your* triggers are, you'll be better able to put coping strategies in place to either avoid them where possible or find healthier ways to deal with your emotions that don't involve food. You can see how Sean and Susan benefited from the process of identifying their triggers in the Food & Mood Journal examples above. It helped them find ways to start overcoming them. Learning how to manage your emotions without food really will be the key to your long-term success. Here is a four-step process that will help you do just that.

1. Pick one emotional trigger to start working on

You might think you can tackle more than one at a time, but most people can't. Start with just one for now. You'll get to the others in due course. Start with the emotional trigger that occurs most frequently for you. For example, if boredom is a trigger now and again but stress is a trigger every day, then choose the latter.

2. Play close attention to your chosen trigger

For example, if you're focusing on stress, try to notice every time it comes up for you going forward and record it in your Food & Mood Journal.

Can you think of occasions when this particular emotional trigger leads you to eat unhealthy or sugary foods? What physical symptoms do you experience? What types of thoughts run through your head at the time? Does it happen at certain times, in certain places or with certain people? Does it affect your eating behaviour at the time or afterwards? What types of food does it make you crave or eat? Does it cause you to overeat?

3. Select a healthy coping strategy

The next step is to choose a healthy coping strategy (that doesn't involve food) and commit to using it each time your trigger comes up. For example, if your trigger is stress, you could try using a deep breathing technique as your healthy coping strategy. So every time you feel stress coming on, practise your deep breathing and repeat this process until your stress levels have reduced. Don't expect the stress to disappear – this is about learning how to manage and tolerate your emotions, not make them go away altogether.

Will these alternative coping strategies be as enjoyable or as effective at soothing you as food? Possibly not, but they will help and give you something else to focus on. Allow yourself time to practise figuring out which coping strategies work best for you. You may find that using a variety of short- and longer-term coping strategies works best. There is a list of healthy coping strategies for a variety of triggers on pages 74–75.

However, in order to truly overcome emotional eating, you also have to learn to tolerate unpleasant feelings and emotions. Which leads me to step 4.

4. Practise tolerating uncomfortable feelings

From a young age we learn to avoid things that make us feel bad. Nobody wants to feel stressed, angry, sad, lonely, rejected or deprived, so we try to numb and distract ourselves from these painful or uncomfortable feelings with things that are not always in our best interests – in this case, food.

The solution? Allow yourself to experience difficult feelings. Much easier said than done, I know, but we often underestimate our ability to cope with and tolerate uncomfortable feelings because we never allow ourselves to sit with them for long enough. We tell ourselves 'I can't stand this feeling', but perhaps you've never even tried. Sometimes we can be so quick to soothe or distract ourselves from uncomfortable feelings that we never really give ourselves the opportunity to process and work through them.

Feelings naturally arise and subside if you let them. Although a feeling may be uncomfortable and unwelcome, it really can't hurt you. But to confirm this for yourself, you have to spend time with your feelings and really allow yourself to feel them.

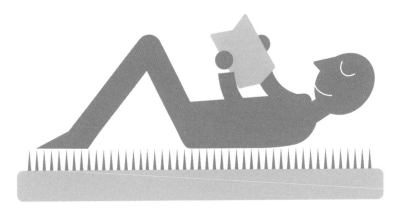

• Do you need additional support? •

If you are having difficulty dealing with particularly painful emotions, perhaps consider seeking individual support from a professional counsellor or therapist.

•Healthy coping strategies for stress •

These strategies also apply to other emotions, such as anger, frustration, etc.

Short-term strategies	Questions to ask yourself	Medium- to long-term strategies
• Deep breathing technique (see page 72) • Go for a walk or run • Talk to a friend or loved one • Play with a child or pet • Do something physically challenging, like gardening or housework • Meditate • Deal with the issue head on	• What are the sources of stress in my life? • Could I be partly responsible for creating or maintaining some of the stress in my life? • Are there sources of stress that I could avoid or limit? • Can I alter the situation or adapt to it? • Do I need to accept the things I cannot change? • Are my current coping strategies healthy or unhealthy? • What can I do in the short term? • What can I do in the long term?	• Better time management • Delegate • Say NO more often • Distance yourself from or challenge the people or relationships that are sources of stress in your life • Engage in stress-busting exercise like walking, running, squash, yoga or tai chi • Read a book on or do a course in stress management, mindfulness or meditation • Consider seeking professional help from a counsellor or therapist

• Healthy coping strategies for other common triggers of emotional eating •

TIREDNESS

Have a stretch, take a short nap, go for a walk, splash cold water on your face, wrap yourself in a warm blanket, drink a hot cup of tea, assess your sleep routine, asses your schedule and adjust where possible. Consider better time management or delegation.

REWARD/PLEASURE SEEKING

If food has become the *only* source of pleasure in your life, it's time to start opening your mind to alternative ways to make yourself feel good. Take a warm bath, indulge in some 'me time', do an activity or hobby you enjoy, read a book or article, have a dance, phone a friend, watch your favourite programme, enjoy a healthy meal or snack, have a daydream, take a nap, do your nails, get your hair done or have a cuddle.

LONELINESS, EMPTINESS, SADNESS

Talk to someone who makes you feel better, look at a favourite photo or cherished memento, do an activity you enjoy (music, gardening, reading, exercise), engage with someone around you, be it a colleague, neighbour or family member, get involved in a social activity, e.g. sports club, walking or book club, take an art or language class, watch a comedy, explore the outdoors, connect with nature.

Consider seeking professional help from a counsellor or therapist if your emotions become unmanageable.

•

How to resist cravings

AS YOU COMPLETE the 10-Day Sugar Challenge you will notice a huge reduction in your physical cravings for sugar and fast-release carbohydrates. However, that's only half the battle because as you well know, your cravings don't just stem from physical hunger – quite often they stem from emotional hunger.

In fact, emotional eating and cravings go hand in hand. A big part of learning how to overcome emotional eating is learning how to resist food cravings. If you're used to succumbing to your food cravings, not giving in to them will take a little bit of practice, but the more often you resist a craving, the less intense and less frequent they'll be in the future.

Every single time you resist a craving, it increases your confidence and strengthens your ability to do it the next time. Conversely, every single time you give in to a craving, it undermines your confidence and weakens your ability to resist your next craving. Bear this in mind the next time you try to tell yourself 'it won't matter just this once'.

Believe me when I say that the more you practise resisting your cravings, the better you'll get at doing it. It helps to view this process as a strengthening exercise – every day you flex your 'I'm not eating sugar' muscle, the stronger and stronger it will get until soon it becomes effortless.

As previously mentioned, reacting to an emotional craving tends to be automatic, instantaneous and virtually mindless. Before you even realise what you're doing, you're halfway through a packet of biscuits. The next time you're hit with a craving, try a technique called **pause and reflect**. This is where you mentally press your internal 'pause button', just like you would on a remote control, and commit to not responding to your craving for 10 minutes (or if that seems unmanageable, try 5 minutes). This will allow you some crucial time to acknowledge what's going on and reflect *before* you act. It also gives you the opportunity to make a different decision. During your pause time, do the following.

Pause and reflect
Label the feeling

Being able to recognise a craving for what it is immediately diminishes its power. Remind yourself: 'This feeling is just a craving. It's strong and uncomfortable, but it's not an emergency and it will pass.'

Remind yourself what you'll gain from learning to resist your craving

Read your benefits list (page 26) and think of all the wonderful benefits you will gain *if* you learn to withstand your cravings. If you don't, you won't. Simple as that.

Make a choice

When you're tempted to eat something you shouldn't, your internal argument ('I want it, but I shouldn't, but I really want it…') creates tension, which makes you feel uncomfortable. You'll be tempted to relieve this tension by choosing to eat. But remember, just as choosing to eat can release this tension, so too can choosing *not* to eat. In other words, you'll instantly feel calmer and more in control the moment you choose *not* to give in to a craving. It's like pulling off a plaster – the quicker you do it, the easier it is.

Distract yourself

Did you know that cravings typically last for 10 to 20 minutes, at which point they start to lose their power and eventually pass? Do yourself a favour and focus your attention on something else entirely for the next 10 minutes or so. Go for a walk, make a call, send an e-mail, paint your nails, do a chore – whatever it takes. You'll be surprised at how quickly your craving diminishes once you choose not to give in to it.

What are you thinking?

Are you having unhelpful or sabotaging thoughts about your ability to handle cravings? If so, reframe your thoughts into more positive, helpful ones. Here's an example.

Negative, unhelpful thought:
I know myself. I won't be able to resist my cravings. They're too strong and I'm too weak.

Positive, helpful thought:
I couldn't resist my cravings in the past, but now is different because I've learned new ways to combat them, both physically (through diet) and emotionally (with new mindset techniques). I'll give these techniques a go because I know I have to learn to overcome cravings if I want look and feel my best.

CHAPTER 6

THE PERFECT BALANCE EATING PLAN

THE 10 GUIDING
PRINCIPLES OF THE
PERFECT BALANCE
EATING PLAN

THE PERFECT
BALANCE EATING
PLAN MEAL
SUGGESTIONS

NEXT
STEPS

NOW THAT YOU HAVE successfully completed the 10-Day Sugar Challenge and learned a variety of new thinking skills, you are ready to transition to a more flexible and long-term eating plan.

The Perfect Balance Eating Plan is a simple and enjoyable food plan that's practical and sustainable for real life. There is no counting calories or points, no weighing food, no magic shakes, pills or bars, just normal, everyday foods eaten in moderation. It provides structure but also flexibility because it can be adapted to suit your individual tastes and lifestyle. As such, the Perfect Balance Eating Plan should suit almost every lifestyle.

It's important for you to know that this is not a diet, it's a way of life. The Perfect Balance Eating Plan simply offers guiding principles that will empower you to make healthy choices for yourself and will enable you to live a low-sugar lifestyle with ease. Essentially, it's an extended and more flexible version of the 10-Day Sugar Challenge so it will be easy to transition to because you're already following many of the key principles.

The main principle behind the Perfect Balance Eating Plan is balance, hence the title. I don't believe in cutting out entire food groups because it's never sustainable for the long term and it often encourages overconsumption of other food groups. For example, if you eliminate carbs from your diet, you're more likely to eat too much protein or fat.

Each macronutrient (protein, carbohydrates, fat) has its place in a balanced diet and offers nutritional value. It's simply about eating the right foods in the right amounts. That's why I call it the Perfect Balance Eating Plan – because it helps you achieve the ideal balance between protein, carbohydrates and healthy fats that will keep your blood sugar levels stable and keep you full and satisfied. It's also loaded with fibre, vitamins, minerals and antioxidants, so you'll get a daily blast of nutrition that will keep you optimally nourished.

The Perfect Balance Eating Plan is designed to steer you away from high-glycemic foods towards low-glycemic foods, which are the best foods for blood sugar control and healthy weight management. I've also got you covered with meal ideas and recipes that largely focus on low- to medium-glycemic foods that will keep your blood sugars stable and stave off cravings. See 'A low-glycemic approach' on page 42 for more information on the glycemic rating system and the benefits of a low-glycemic diet.

The Perfect Balance Eating Plan is designed to:

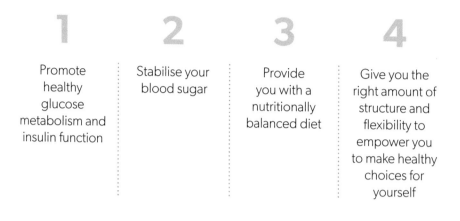

1 Promote healthy glucose metabolism and insulin function

2 Stabilise your blood sugar

3 Provide you with a nutritionally balanced diet

4 Give you the right amount of structure and flexibility to empower you to make healthy choices for yourself

As a result of the above, the Perfect Balance Eating Plan will:

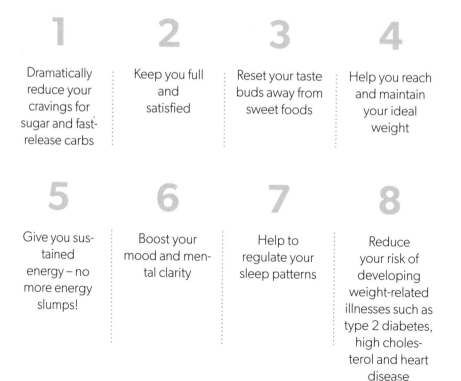

1 Dramatically reduce your cravings for sugar and fast-release carbs

2 Keep you full and satisfied

3 Reset your taste buds away from sweet foods

4 Help you reach and maintain your ideal weight

5 Give you sustained energy – no more energy slumps!

6 Boost your mood and mental clarity

7 Help to regulate your sleep patterns

8 Reduce your risk of developing weight-related illnesses such as type 2 diabetes, high cholesterol and heart disease

So how does it work? To follow the Perfect Balance Eating Plan, all you need to do is follow the **10 guiding principles** in this chapter. These principles are the building blocks for living a low-sugar lifestyle and having a healthy and balanced relationship with all types of food, including sugar! They've been designed to be simple and straightforward so that you can easily incorporate them into your lifestyle. Sticking to the principles will give you the tools to control your cravings, appetite, weight, energy and overall health and well-being.

•

The 10 guiding principles of the Perfect Balance Eating Plan

10 guiding principles

1. Limit your intake of added sugars.

2. Include protein with every meal and snack.

3. Favour slow-release carbs.

4. Get the balance right at mealtimes.

5. Eat healthy fats.

6. Eat at regular intervals.

7. Get your five a day (minimum!).

8. Eat natural, minimally processed foods.

9. Limit caffeine.

10. Alcohol in moderation.

1. Limit your intake of added sugars

In order to limit your sugar intake going forward, you'll need to become aware of added sugars. Added sugars refers to all types of sugars that are *added* to food by the manufacturer, the cook or the consumer as well as sugars that are naturally present in honey, syrups, fruit juices and fruit concentrates. Added sugars are sometimes referred to as 'free sugars'.

Added sugars do not include the sugars that are *naturally present* in foods such as whole fruit, vegetables, milk, grains and other plant-based foods like legumes and nuts. All of these foods can be eaten in moderation on the Perfect Balance Eating Plan.

Essentially, following this principle means not adding any form of sugar to your food and drinks and limiting your intake of packaged foods and drinks that contain added sugars. Doing so will enable you to live a low-sugar lifestyle, which for most people is a lot more feasible and sustainable than a no-sugar lifestyle.

Checking labels for sugar content is the simplest way to assess how much sugar is contained in a packaged food or drink. In Chapter 7 I will teach you how to recognise all the forms of sugar on food and drink labels and how to easily work out how much sugar is contained in a food or drink.

For optimal health, the World Health Organization currently recommends that sugars should make up less than 5% of our total energy intake per day. This is equivalent to around 25 grams (approx. 6 teaspoons) of sugar per day for an adult with a normal body mass index (BMI). Note that this is a recommended daily *limit*, not a *target*. Following the principles behind the Perfect Balance Eating Plan will ensure your sugar intake stays well below the recommended daily limit.

2. Include protein with every meal and snack

You're already familiar with this principle from the 10-Day Sugar Challenge and have probably felt the benefit of it already. Including protein with every meal and snack is important for a number of reasons. Firstly, when you eat protein alongside a carbohydrate, it helps to slow down the rate at which the carbohydrate breaks down into glucose and hits your bloodstream. For example, adding chicken or meat to pasta will slow down the rate at which the pasta is broken down into glucose and absorbed by the body. Essentially, pairing protein with carbohydrates will help to keep your blood glucose and insulin levels stable, so you're less likely to have cravings or energy dips throughout the day.

Protein also helps you stay fuller for longer, which is good news for weight management. But remember, when it comes to a healthy protein intake, both quality and quantity are key. The Perfect Balance Eating Plan is not a high-protein diet, nor does it encourage a high intake of animal protein and/or saturated fats. On the contrary, too much protein in the diet (particularly animal protein) can lead to a situation in which minerals are released from the bones to counteract the acidity of the blood. This is a natural occurrence when too much protein is eaten and can lead to reduced bone density. In addition, having to break down large amounts of protein can put a strain on the kidneys in sensitive individuals.

Following the guidelines below will ensure that each of your meals contains a healthy quantity of protein and is well balanced against other nutrients that are required for optimal health and weight management.

PROTEIN PORTION GUIDELINES

Instead of weighing your food, I recommend using simple visual guidelines to help get your portion sizes right. As you've already learned, the portion of protein you should aim to eat at main meals should be roughly the size of the palm of your hand.

However, consuming a palm-sized portion of protein at breakfast isn't always practical or even necessary. The breakfast suggestions and recipes I've given you all contain adequate amounts of protein to ensure you'll be eating a balanced breakfast.

Similarly, all of the snack suggestions incorporate just enough protein (approx. half a palm-sized portion) to help keep your blood sugar stable and reduce hunger and cravings.

ANIMAL VS. PLANT PROTEIN

By now you know that the type of protein you eat is just as important as the quantity. Many people have a tendency to consume too many animal sources of protein, such as red meat and dairy, which is not healthful. For optimal health, I recommend you eat more plant protein and fish and less red meat and dairy.

Beans, lentils, nuts, seeds and quinoa are good sources of plant protein. They are highly nutritious foods that contain quality protein, complex carbohydrates, healthy fats and fibre as well as countless vitamins and minerals. As such, they should feature regularly as part of a healthy and balanced diet. The meal suggestions and recipes will give you lots of ways to incorporate these foods into your diet.

Personally, I strive for a 50–50 balance between animal protein and plant protein. Play around and see what ratio works best for you.

The main sources of animal and plant-based protein are:
- **Animal protein:** Meat, fish, poultry, eggs, dairy
- **Plant protein:** Beans, lentils, nuts, seeds, tofu, tempeh, quinoa

3. Favour slow-release carbs

Many people believe that avoiding carbs is the key to achieving successful weight management. However, carbohydrates are an important part of a healthy diet. They provide your body with the fuel it needs for physical activity and proper organ function and help to keep your mood in balance.

However, problems arise when we consume *too much* of the *wrong types* of carbohydrates. Eating the appropriate amounts of the right types of carbohydrate is actually essential for good health and weight management, which is why they have their rightful place on the Perfect Balance Eating Plan. When choosing a carbohydrate-rich food at mealtimes, favour slow- or medium-release carbohydrates over fast-release carbohydrates. This is because not all carbs are created equal – see the table on the next page for a list of slow-, medium- and fast-release carbohydrates.

Let's do a quick recap to make sure you are fully clued in about carbs. As previously mentioned, carbohydrates can be divided into two main categories: fast-release carbs and slow-release carbs.

Fast-release carbohydrates break down into glucose very quickly, giving us a sugar high followed by a sugar low. When we consume these easily digested, 'fast-releasing' carbohydrates, sugar is rapidly released into the bloodstream, providing a burst of energy. This sudden sugar rush is too much for the body to make use of, so any excess is then turned into fat, creating a sudden drop in blood sugar. This will leave you feeling tired, hungry and craving yet more carbs or sugar to perk yourself back up.

Fast-release carbohydrates tend to be refined and highly processed foods with a low fibre content and little nutritional value. They generally have a high glycemic rating (see page 42 for more information).

Slow-release carbohydrates, on the other hand, break down into sugar more slowly, so we get a slow and steady release of energy without spiking blood sugar or insulin levels. Slow-release carbohydrates tend to be either whole foods, e.g. vegetables, or wholegrain foods, e.g. oats. They are naturally high in fibre so they keep you fuller for longer, boost digestion and supply you with a range of vitamins and minerals. In addition, fibre slows down the rate at which carbohydrates break down into sugar. Slow-release carbohydrates generally have a low to medium glycemic rating (see page 42).

Fast-release carbohydrates	Slow- or medium-release carbohydrates
Bagels	Beans
Biscuits	Brown rice
Breakfast bars	Bulgur wheat
Cake	Lentils
Chips	Millet
Chocolate	Most whole fruits and vegetables**
Crisps	Oats
Dried fruit	Pearl barley
Fruit juices	Quinoa
Honey	Sweet potatoes
Ice cream	Whole wheat pasta
Jam	Wholegrain bread
Jellies	
Muffins	
Pastry or baked goods	
Pizza	
Refined cereals	
Refined crackers	
Scones	
Soft drinks	
Sweets	
White bread	
White flour foods, e.g. scones	
White pasta or noodles	
White potatoes*	
White rice	

*White potatoes are considered to be fast-releasing carbohydrates. However, if you limit yourself to modest portions, they can be eaten in moderation as part of a balanced diet. Boiled potatoes with their skins on are a better choice then baked or chipped potatoes.

**See the 'Carbohydrates better choice guide' on page 87 for advice on the best fruit choices.

CARBOHYDRATE PORTION GUIDE

- **1 slice of wholegrain bread = 1 portion**
- **1 medium potato (6–7.5cm diameter) = 1 portion**
- **½ cup oats (approx. 40g) = 1 portion**
- **½ cup (approx. 3 heaped tablespoons) cooked rice, quinoa, barley, pasta, etc. = 1 portion**
- **2 oatcakes or rye crispbreads = ½ portion (e.g. as a snack or a side)**
- **4 oatcakes or rye crispbreads = 1 portion**

I recommend eating between two and four portions of carbohydrate-rich food (preferably slow-releasing) per day depending on your activity level and whether or not you need to lose weight.

ENERGY MODIFICATIONS BASED ON ACTIVITY LEVEL

If you have a very active lifestyle, work at a physically demanding job and/or regularly participate in high-intensity physical activity or exercise, you may need to consume four or more portions of carbohydrate-rich food per day.

In terms of plate ratios, your portion of carbohydrate-rich food may take up a little more than one-quarter of the plate (such as two-thirds of a cup of cooked rice) and/or you can afford to include more starchy vegetables as part of your vegetable allowance.

Please note that these guidelines are estimates only. If you find that you need more carbohydrates to maintain activity, adjust your needs.

WEIGHT LOSS MODIFICATIONS

If you need to lose weight, limit yourself to two or three portions of carbohydrate-rich foods per day until you reach a healthy weight range. This may mean omitting a portion of carbohydrate-rich food from one meal per day and just having protein and vegetables for that meal, e.g. a tuna salad or steak with cauliflower mash.

FRUIT AND VEGETABLES

When we think of carbohydrates we tend to think of starchy foods such as bread or pasta. We forget that fruits and vegetables also contain carbohydrates.

In general, most fruits and vegetables can be classed as slow-release carbohydrates. However, some fruits and vegetables contain a higher amount of fast-releasing sugars than others and so need to be eaten in moderation. These include starchy vegetables such as potatoes, parsnips, swedes and yams and sweet fruits such as bananas, grapes, pineapple or mango.

The table on the next page will help guide you in terms of which carbohydrates (including fruits and vegetables) to eat more often and which to eat less often and in moderate amounts.

CARBOHYDRATES BETTER CHOICE GUIDE

	Grain- or seed-based foods	Vegetables	Fruit

Great choice
The slow-release carbohydrates in this category are ideal choices because they are relatively low-glycemic foods, which means they will keep your blood sugar levels stable so that you'll feel fuller and energised for longer.
	Amaranth
	Bulgur wheat
	Millet
	Oats
	Pearl barley
	Quinoa
		Asparagus
		Bean sprouts
		Broccoli
		Brussels sprouts
		Cabbage
		Cauliflower
		Celery
		Courgettes
		Cucumbers
		Fennel
		Green beans
		Green leafy
		  vegetables
		Kale
		Leeks
		Lettuce
		Mangetout
		Mushrooms
		Onions (all types)
		Peppers
		Rocket
		Runner beans
		Spinach
		Watercress
			Apples
			Apricots (fresh)
			Avocado*
			Blackberries
			Blueberries
			Cranberries
			 (fresh)
			Gooseberries
			Grapefruit
			Lemon and lime
			Pears
			Plums
			Raspberries
			Strawberries
			Tomatoes
			
			* Limit to two
			   per week

Good choice
The foods at this level will trigger a moderate glycemic response, which means they will raise blood sugar levels at a reasonably steady rate provided they're eaten in moderate amounts.
  The foods in this category are nutritious foods but still need to be eaten in moderate amounts.
	Brown rice
	Couscous
	Soba noodles
	Whole wheat
	  pasta or noodles
	Wholegrain bread
		Aubergines
		Beetroot
		Butternut squash
		Carrots
		Parsnips
		Peas
		Pumpkins
		Swedes
		Sweet potatoes
		Yams
			Cherries
			Grapes
			Mangoes
			Melons
			Nectarines
			Papayas
			Peaches
			Pineapples
			Tangerines

Adequate choice *Most of the foods in this category contain fast-release carbohydrates, so they will raise blood sugar levels fast and provide only short-term energy. Although the fruit and vegetables in this category do offer nutritional value, they need to be eaten in strict moderation to maintain blood sugar balance.*	Egg or rice noodles White pasta White rice	Sweetcorn White potatoes	Bananas Dates Dried fruit Figs Fruit juices Prunes

4. Get the balance right at mealtimes

A balanced diet starts with getting the balance right at mealtimes. A nutritionally balanced meal is one that contains the correct balance (i.e. proportions) of protein, carbohydrates and fat and includes plenty of vegetables for added fibre and nutrition.

Eating the proper ratio of protein, carbohydrates and fats at mealtimes keeps blood sugar stable, helps maintain physical and emotional balance, stops food cravings and sustains energy levels. You're probably comfortable with and have already felt the benefit of this principle from following the 10-Day Sugar Challenge.

Here's how to divide you plate for a balanced meal:

- One-quarter of your meal should consist of **protein-rich food(s)** such as fish, eggs, meat, tofu or a serving of beans or lentils. You can combine various proteins if you wish.
- Another quarter of your meal should contain **carbohydrate-rich food(s)** such as brown rice, potatoes, quinoa, bulgur wheat, wholegrain bread, whole wheat pasta, oats, pearl barley, etc.
- The remaining half of your meal should be made up of vegetables. At least half of these should be **non-starchy** vegetables (see the guide on page 87).

Guidelines on how to incorporate the right amount of healthy fats in your diet are given in the next section.

Note: There isn't a natural division between protein and carbs in plant foods. They all have some of both in various quantities. For example, beans and lentils contain both protein and carbohydrates. You should count beans and lentils as your protein portion if you haven't already met your protein intake with other protein foods and count any remaining servings of beans and lentils you eat as part of your carbohydrate portion. In fact, including beans or lentils as part of your carbohydrate portion would lower the overall carbohydrate load of your meal, which is particularly good for weight management.

The grain quinoa also contains a good mix of carbs and protein. I recommend counting quinoa as part of your carb portion. Doing so will also lower the overall carbohydrate load of your meal.

5. Eat healthy fats

Since the early 1980s, health experts have preached that a low-fat diet is the key to maintaining a healthy weight, managing heart health and preventing various health problems. As consumers we've completely bought into the notion that low-fat food equals healthy food.

A walk down any supermarket aisle will confirm our continuing obsession with low-fat and diet foods. The shelves are piled high with low-fat this, no-fat that and fat-free the other. We're bombarded with 'guilt-free' options, from low-fat ice cream, biscuits and cakes to fat-free yoghurts and cereals. Yet while the number of low-fat options continues to expand, so too do our waistlines and obesity rates. We spend millions of euros every year on diet food, yet we're in the midst of an obesity epidemic. Clearly, low-fat diet foods are not delivering on their 'stay slim and healthy' promises.

The problem is that we have become so used to hearing about the evils of fats that we assume all types of fat are bad and tar them all with the same brush. I hear so many people say that they'd feel better about eating a handful of low-fat biscuits than a handful of nuts, which is ludicrous. The reality is that not all fats are created equal. And despite what you've been told, fat isn't always the villain in the waistline wars. The answer isn't cutting fat out of your diet: it's simply eating more of the healthy fats and eating less of the unhealthy ones.

Our bodies actually *need* certain types of fat in order to function well. For example, essential fatty acids (EFAs) are necessary fats that humans can't synthesise, so they must be obtained through diet. There are two families of EFAs: omega-3 and omega-6. Omega-9 is necessary yet 'non-essential' because the body can manufacture a modest amount on its own, provided other EFAs are present.

There is a lot of conflicting information out there on fats and even a big variance in opinion from one health expert to the next. In the interest of keeping things simple and clear, here's my advice on fats.

BALANCE YOUR OMEGA-6 TO OMEGA-3 RATIO

In general, most people tend to consume a lot more omega-6 fats (e.g. sunflower oil, corn oil) than omega-3 fats (e.g. oily fish, chia seed), which is not ideal for health. Eating too much omega-6 fats and not enough omega-3 fats contributes to inflammation in the body, which is a major driver of disease.

It's important to consume omega-6 fats and omega-3 fats in a healthy balance, and as close to a 1:1 ratio as possible, although a ratio of 2:1 or even 3:1 of omega-6 to omega-3 is probably more realistic and achievable for most people.

To ensure you are getting enough omega-3 fats in your diet, have 1 tablespoon of ground seeds per day *or* 1 tablespoon of cold-pressed seed oil per day. The seeds and oils I recommend are the ones that are high in omega-3, such as flax, hemp and chia.

In addition, you should eat oily fish (e.g. salmon, trout, sardines, mackerel, tuna), which are high in omega-3 fats, two to three times per week. If you don't eat fish, consider taking a fish oil or krill oil supplement to boost your omega-3 intake.

Please note that many foods contain a mixture of different fats.

Omega-3 benefits

Extensive research indicates that omega-3 fats reduce inflammation, which helps to prevent inflammatory diseases like heart disease and arthritis. In addition to warding off inflammation, research suggests that omega-3s may also:

- Improve cholesterol by lowering triglycerides and elevating HDL ('good' cholesterol)

- Improve artery health by helping to reduce plaque build-up

- Safeguard mental health and enhance brain function

- Improve joint health by reducing joint stiffness associated with arthritis

- Alleviate symptoms related to skin conditions like eczema and psoriasis

- Support bowel health by reducing inflammation of the bowels

- Reduce the symptoms of PMS and menstrual pain

EAT SATURATED FATS IN MODERATION

For decades we've been told that saturated fat from animal products such as meat, eggs, cream and cheese raises blood cholesterol levels and increases the risk of heart disease and stroke. However, recent studies are now challenging this long-held belief, concluding that people who eat moderate amounts of naturally occurring saturated fat do not experience more cardiovascular disease than those who eat less.

Does this mean we can eat as much saturated fat as we want? I'm afraid not. Eating a diet high in saturated fat is still not good for your overall health or your waistline. Most of our saturated fat intake comes from naturally occurring fats found in meat and dairy.

If you choose to consume dairy, eat natural, full-fat versions of dairy but in moderate amounts. That way you're likely to feel more full and satisfied by what you've eaten, even if it's a smaller portion. In addition, you'll be eating a food in its whole, natural, unadulterated state, which is best all round.

Where red meat is concerned, choose lean cuts and limit your consumption to no more than twice per week.

AVOID HYDROGENATED AND TRANS FATS

The fats you want to avoid altogether are the artificial man-made fats that our bodies don't know how to process. These are known as trans fats or hydrogenated fats.

When the molecules of polyunsaturated fats are altered by food processing (called hydrogenation) or frying at high temperatures, they can no longer benefit the body and are called trans fats. In recent years, trans fats have received a lot of bad press from being linked to a host of health problems, from heart disease to diabetes. As a result, manufacturers now make a point of advertising products as 'trans fat-free'.

But don't be fooled. The food industry has been busy perfecting another man-made replacement in the form of interesterified fats, which appear to have similar health effects. These types of fats are often found in margarine, shortening, chips, fried chicken, baked goods, biscuits, pastries, crisps and crackers.

To avoid these artificial fats, look out for the following words on ingredients lists: **partially hydrogenated oils, interesterified fats or oil, high stearate or stearic-rich fats**. Your best bet is to buy whole foods and cook or bake from scratch.

Which oils are best for cooking and cold uses?

When cooking at high temperatures it's best to use oils with a higher smoke point, such as cold-pressed vegetable oils, virgin coconut oil or butter. For cold uses, extra virgin olive oil, hemp oil or flaxseed oil are excellent choices.

However, recent studies on olive oil show that despite having fatty acids with double bonds, you can still use it for medium-heat cooking, as it is fairly resistant to heat. When I'm gently sweating veg I'm happy to use olive oil, as the heat never reaches a perilous point. If you want to keep cooking temperatures down, you can always add a little water to your pan as you cook to maintain a moderate temperature that won't denature your oil.

6. Eat at regular intervals

Eating at regular intervals is a crucial element of the Perfect Balance Eating Plan. If you leave long gaps between meals, your blood sugar levels will drop too low, leaving you weak and ravenous. You are much more likely to over-eat and/or choose the wrong type of foods when you are too hungry and have low blood sugar. As you know, the main aim of this eating plan is to keep your blood sugar levels stable throughout the day.

Stable blood sugar levels = lasting energy, reduced sugar and carb cravings, better mood and better concentration

In order to maintain stable blood sugar levels, you will need to eat the right types of foods in the right amounts at the right time. Following the principles of the Perfect Balance Eating Plan makes it easy for you to do this and ensures you'll have balanced blood sugar levels throughout the day.

Fuelling up frequently ensures that there is a constant and steady supply of glucose in the bloodstream and keeps your metabolism revved.

TOP TIP

ALWAYS HAVE HEALTHY SNACKS

CLOSE TO HAND SO YOU HAVE NO

EXCUSE WHEN TEMPTATION STRIKES.

SEE PAGE 107 FOR HEALTHY SNACK

SUGGESTIONS.

DON'T GO LONGER THAN THREE HOURS WITHOUT EATING SOMETHING. THREE MAIN MEALS PER DAY PLUS A MID-MORNING AND MID-AFTERNOON SNACK IS IDEAL.

HIGH BLOOD SUGAR

NORMAL BLOOD SUGAR

LOW BLOOD SUGAR

BLOOD SUGAR ROLLERCOASTER = ENERGY ROLLERCOASTER

Here is a sample menu with sample timings.

BREAKFAST – 8.00am
Poached egg on rye toast

MID-MORNING SNACK – 11.00am
Natural yoghurt topped with fruit and a sprinkle of seeds

LUNCH – 1.00pm
Lentil and vegetable soup + 2 oatcakes with cheese or hummus

MID-AFTERNOON SNACK – 4.00pm
Sliced apple with peanut butter

DINNER – 7.00pm
Shepherd's pie with veg

7. Get your five a day (at least!) •

Besides helping you banish sugar and carb cravings, the Perfect Balance Eating Plan will also help you develop healthy habits that will stand to you now and well into the future. Not only does it strike the perfect balance between protein, carbohydrates and essential fats, it's also loaded with fibre, vitamins, minerals and antioxidants so that you'll get a daily blast of nutrition for optimal health and disease prevention.

You'll also glow from the inside out. Many clients report a significant boost in skin radiance when they increase their fruit and vegetable intake to optimal levels.

Consuming the right amount of fruit and vegetables is an essential part of the Perfect Balance Eating Plan because fruit and veg provide a large proportion of the nutrients you need to look and feel your best.

• WHY EAT MORE FRUIT AND VEGETABLES? •

Extensive research suggests that eating a minimum of five portions of fruit and vegetables per day may help to protect us from a variety of diet-related diseases.

• WHAT ARE THE HEALTH BENEFITS IF I EAT ENOUGH FRUIT AND VEGETABLES? •

1
You have less chance of developing obesity and type 2 diabetes.

2
You have less chance of developing cardio-vascular disease.

3
You have less chance of developing some cancers, such as bowel and lung cancer.

Fruit and vegetables also:

1
Contain lots of fibre, which helps to keep your bowels healthy. Adequate fibre in the diet can also help to control cholesterol levels and keep blood sugar levels stable.

2
Are rich in a host of vitamins, minerals and antioxidants, which boost our immunity and help to protect us from illness.

3
Provide antioxidant vitamins like beta caro-tene, vitamin C and vitamin E, which boost skin radiance and help to prevent premature ageing.

TOP TIP: EAT A RAINBOW EVERY DAY

To maximise the amount and variety of vitamins and minerals in your diet, try picking a 'rainbow' of different coloured fruits and vegetables to eat every day, from dark leafy greens to bright citrus fruits and every colour in between.

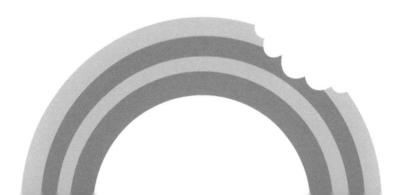

Ideally, limit your fruit intake to two portions per day. This is enough to provide you with plenty of the nutrients that fruit has to offer without throwing your blood sugar balance off kilter. The rest of your intake should come from vegetables.

You should also focus more on low-glycemic (i.e. low-sugar) fruits and vegetables. See the table on page 87 for a guide to the best choice of fruit and veg. High-glycemic fruits such as bananas and dates should be viewed as treat foods and/or used to provide natural sweetness for occasional baking or desserts.

• TO JUICE OR NOT TO JUICE? •

When a fruit is juiced, the fibre and pulp are left behind during the juicing process. It's the fibre in fruit that helps slow down the absorption of sugar and also keeps our bowel and gut healthy, so glugging your way through a glass of fruit juice can give you a sugar high but then a subsequent sugar crash. And remember, any excess sugar that the body can't use gets stored as fat. End of.

In general it's best to stick to whole fruits, so eat an orange whole as opposed to orange juice. If juices appeal to you, make sure to only consume a very small quantity and ideally dilute it with some water. Juices that combine both fruit and vegetables are also a better option than fruit juice alone. For example, carrot, apple, lemon and ginger juice is a nicely balanced juice combination.

8. Choose natural foods when possible and minimally processed foods when not

It goes without saying that the very best food comes from nature and not a laboratory. By sticking to whole, natural foods that haven't been genetically altered, you're eating foods that speak the same language as your body and therefore can be digested and absorbed effectively. You also know exactly what you're putting into your body and won't have to worry about trying to interpret misleading food labels.

Unfortunately, many highly processed foods are laden with sugar, artificial sweeteners, salt, flavour enhancers, factory-created fats, colourings and preservatives. But the trouble isn't just what's been added – it's also what's been taken away.

Processed foods are often stripped of nutrients designed by nature to protect your heart, such as soluble fibre, antioxidants and essential fats. We also don't benefit from the living enzymes and natural nutrients that fresh food normally contains, which aids digestion and nutrient absorption.

Of course, not all processed foods are unhealthy. Cheese, rice, tinned lentils, nut butter and porridge oats have all been processed in some way before they reach supermarket shelves, but they receive *minimal processing* and thus aren't a cause for concern.

Most health professionals will recommend limiting the amount of processed foods in your diet, which is what you want to strive for. But with the abundance of processed foods available in modern society, this can be challenging. The following rule of thumb is probably a more realistic and achievable goal for most people:

Choose natural foods when possible
and minimally processed foods when not.

For the most part, the closer a food is to its natural form, the healthier it is. The more processed it is, the less nutritious it will be. Always opt for unprocessed or minimally processed foods where possible. Another good rule of thumb is that if a food label has a long list of ingredients you don't recognise or can't pronounce, then it's probably best left on the shelf.

TRY TO CONSUME BETWEEN FIVE AND EIGHT PORTIONS OF FRUIT AND VEGETABLES EVERY DAY FOR OPTIMAL HEALTH AND DISEASE PREVENTION. THIS MAY SOUND LIKE A LOT, BUT THE MEAL SUGGESTIONS AND RECIPES IN THIS BOOK WILL MAKE IT SURPRISINGLY EASY FOR YOU TO GET YOUR 'FIVE A DAY' (AND LIKELY MORE) WITH LITTLE EFFORT.

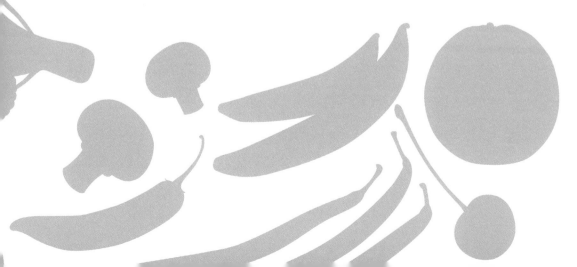

Ready-made meals – good or bad?

If you're time starved, you may be tempted to take the easy option and go for ready-made meals at dinnertime. No prepping, no cooking, no washing up, just two minutes in the microwave and hey presto, dinner is served.

Opting for a ready-made meal now and then won't harm your health, but if you regularly rely on them, you could be unknowingly sabotaging your health and your weight. Here's why.

Most ready-made meals are:

High in fat and calories: For example, one serving of a well-known supermarket brand of chicken korma and rice contains 38.4g of fat – that's as much fat as as you'd find in three chocolate bars.

High in salt: Many ready-made meals, such as cottage pie or chicken chow mein, contain up to 3 grams of salt – that's half your recommended daily intake of salt in just one serving.

High in sugar: A well-known supermarket brand of sweet and sour chicken with rice contains 20g of sugar per serving – that's equivalent to 5 teaspoons of sugar in your dinner.

High in flavour enhancers, including MSG: Many packet soups and noodle dishes contain this artificial flavour, which is linked to a variety of health issues, including headaches, palpitations, asthma and eczema.

• ARE LOW-FAT OR DIET FOODS A BETTER CHOICE? •

When fat is removed from a food, it generally has to be replaced with something else in order to retain flavour. More often than not, fat is replaced with sugar and/or artificial sweeteners. For example, a low-fat yoghurt will often contain two to three times more sugar than a full-fat yoghurt.

What's more, low-fat or fat-free foods often leave you hungry and craving more. One reason for this is that fat is filling and satisfying. For example, you're more likely to feel satisfied after one tub of full-fat yoghurt than one tub of low-fat yoghurt. In addition, fat slows down the release of sugars from foods, which keeps blood sugar levels from rising too rapidly. Using the yoghurt example again, the sugar in a low-fat yoghurt would enter the bloodstream quicker than the sugar from a full-fat yoghurt, which can lead to a blood sugar spike.

Stick to foods in their natural form as much as possible and be mindful of portion sizes when it comes to those that are naturally high in fat.

9. Limit caffeine

Caffeine (found in coffee, tea and energy drinks) acts as a stimulant in the body. It revs up stress hormones such as adrenalin and cortisol, which can interfere with blood sugar balance and in turn lead to cravings for sugar and carbs. Think about it: how often do you have a tea or coffee without looking for a biscuit or something sweet to go with it?

Ideally, I recommend that you avoid caffeinated beverages altogether, particularly if you are sensitive to caffeine. But if you don't feel the need to give up tea or coffee altogether, then limit yourself to no more than two cups of either tea or coffee per day. Avoid energy drinks, colas or any type of soft drink altogether, including diet versions.

The best way to cut your caffeine intake is to wean yourself off caffeinated beverages one cup at a time, a few days at a time. Try alternating every second cup of tea or coffee with either a decaf version or a herbal tea. If you choose to drink decaf coffee, opt for organic decaf that is free from chemical solvents, which are often used to extract the caffeine. Remember, though, that if you continue to drink decaf coffee, you will still have a taste and desire for coffee, which is self-defeating in some ways.

IS CAFFEINE MAKING YOU STRESSED?

If you're prone to anxiety or stress, I strongly recommend that you avoid caffeine altogether, as caffeine sets off a stress response in the body every time you consume it. As previously mentioned, caffeine stimulates your adrenal glands to make adrenalin, which sets the stress response in motion, causing tense muscles, elevated blood sugar and an increased heart and breathing rate.

You may feel mentally sharper for a little while because your brain is high on adrenalin, but it's a jittery energy that's short lived. An hour later, you're likely to feel tired but wired as the caffeine wears off but the stress hormones are left circulating in your system. As your body comes down off the adrenalin, you'll feel the drop in terms of fatigue, irritability and headache and will likely reach for another cup to perk yourself up again.

If you constantly keep your body on a caffeine high, you're constantly keeping your body in 'stress mode'. Sooner or later it starts to take a toll on your body, particularly if you already have multiple sources of stress in your life. And even though most people think caffeine makes them mentally sharper, studies clearly demonstrate that in fact, the opposite is true.

At least nine out of 10 of my clients report that they feel calmer, less stressed and are sleeping better as soon as they cut out the caffeine. Try it and see for yourself.

10. Alcohol in moderation •

If you want to maintain blood sugar balance, keep your cravings under control and your weight down, you'll need to limit your consumption of alcohol.

Alcohol breaks down into sugar, which raises blood glucose levels rapidly and stimulates appetite and cravings. Have you ever noticed that you eat more when you consume alcohol with a meal? Or that you crave certain foods while you are drinking, or perhaps the next day?

Not only does alcohol send your blood sugar levels soaring and stimulate your appetite, but it also weakens your resolve, which can undermine all your good efforts. On top of that, regular alcohol consumption inhibits fat loss and encourages weight gain, particularly fat around the middle, so you can see why it's in your interests to limit your intake.

Having said that, alcohol can be enjoyed as part of a healthy and balanced lifestyle, provided that it's taken in moderation. I suggest that you drink alcohol no more than three times per week (preferably less) and that you limit yourself to no more than two units of alcohol per sitting. Note that this is a recommended *limit*, not a *target*. Less is best, especially while you're getting used to your new way of eating.

WHAT IS A STANDARD DRINK?

In Ireland, a standard drink has about 10 grams of pure alcohol in it. In the UK, a standard drink, also called a unit of alcohol, has about 8 grams of pure alcohol.

Here are some examples of a standard drink:
- **A pub measure of spirits (35.5ml)**
- **A small glass of wine (12.5% ABV)**
- **A half pint of normal beer**
- **A bottle of wine at 12.5% alcohol contains about seven standard drinks**

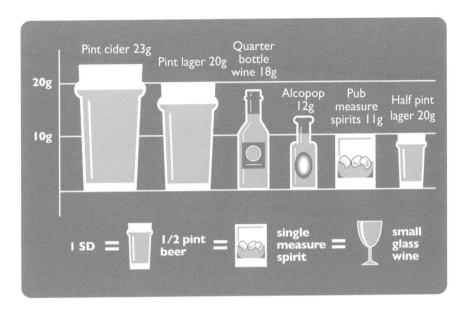

Remember, drink measures aren't always the same. What you get in a bar or restaurant and what you pour for yourself at home could be very different.

These recommended weekly limits don't apply to teenagers or to people who are pregnant, ill, run-down or on medication.

WHAT ARE THE BEST OPTIONS?

A dry wine is your best choice when it comes to alcohol, or else spirits drunk neat or with soda water and perhaps a squeeze of fresh lemon or lime.

Beer and cider have the highest carbohydrate content, so they are not good choices.

Alcohol and cancer risk

Did you know that heavy or regular alcohol consumption increases the risk of developing several forms of cancer? Based on extensive reviews of research studies, there is a strong scientific consensus on an association between drinking alcohol and several types of cancer. The research evidence indicates that the more alcohol a person drinks (particularly the more alcohol a person drinks regularly over time), the higher his or her risk of developing an alcohol-associated cancer.

The Perfect Balance Eating Plan meal suggestions

NOW THAT YOU know the guiding principles behind the Perfect Balance Eating Plan, it's time to show you how to put these principles into practice in a way that's appealing yet practical.

The selection of suggested meal and snack options provides a springboard to encourage you to think for yourself when deciding what you should eat at mealtimes and how to combine the right foods in the right ratios. They'll provide inspiration as to how you can best apply the principles to your own diet and lifestyle.

Incorporating the Perfect Balance Eating Plan principles into your lifestyle will require a bit of extra thought and planning at first, but once you get into the swing of things, you'll realise just how easy and enjoyable it is and it will become second nature.

Remember, these meal suggestions are ideas only. Feel free to use the guidelines and come up with your own creations.

• Breakfast suggestions •

CEREAL-BASED BREAKFAST

Porridge oats (cooked or raw): Made with water or a milk of your choice. Add some chopped nuts or milled seeds to add protein and healthy fats. To sweeten, try cinnamon and/or fruit such as grated apple or berries.

Granola: Most store-bought brands of granola are high in sugar, as they're loaded with dried fruit. You may be able to find a sugar-free granola with no dried fruit at your local health food store. If so, choose one that's oat based with plenty of nuts and seeds or add your own. I recommend you make your own granola – see page 148 for my recipe. Serve with milk or natural yoghurt and top with a fruit of your choice.

Wholegrain cereal: Good options include cereals made from one or a combination of different wholegrains, including whole wheat, buckwheat, rye, millet and quinoa. Just be sure to check the label for sugar and fibre content (see the guidelines below).

Cereal guidelines:
• Add 1–2 tablespoons of chopped nuts or milled seeds to your cereal to add protein and healthy fats.
• Sweeten your cereal with low-glycemic fruit such as apple, pear or berries for added vitamins and fibre.

- Try adding spices such as cinnamon, nutmeg or ginger for extra flavour.
- Only choose store-bought cereal, muesli or granola with less than 6g sugar per 100g and at least 7g of fibre per 100g.

COOKED BREAKFASTS

Eggs: One or two eggs cooked as you wish served with a slice of wholegrain toast or a couple of oatcakes. For extra vitamins and fibre, add some veggies, such as grilled tomato, mushroom, spinach, avocado or asparagus.

Smoked salmon or cooked meats are also an option, but processed meats such as bacon or sausage should only ever be eaten in strict moderation, as they are high in saturated fat and preservatives.

Fish: Smoked salmon or haddock or kippers served on a bed of steamed spinach drizzled with olive oil.

Pancakes: Try my power pancake recipe on page 151. It's super filling due to its high protein content.

ON-THE-MOVE BREAKFASTS

Smoothies: A smoothie is a good option for an on-the-go breakfast. Ideally use low-glycemic fruit such as berries and add some protein and healthy fats with ground nuts or milled seeds such as flax, chia or hemp seed. Natural whole milk yoghurt adds protein too or you can use a variety of different milk options. See page 152 for my supercharger smoothie recipe.

Nut butter: Try a couple of teaspoons of sugar-free peanut butter or almond/cashew nut butter spread on a couple of oatcakes or a slice of wholegrain bread or toast.

Yoghurt: Three tablespoons of natural yoghurt topped with fruit and a tablespoon of milled seeds makes for a speedy but nutritious breakfast. Whole milk natural yoghurt is ideal as low-fat natural yoghurt can be a little bitter and is less filling. If you choose a probiotic yoghurt you'll also be boosting your digestive health.

Nuts: A palmful of nuts with a piece of fruit is a fairly good on-the-run breakfast, albeit less substantial than the other options.

Breakfast ideas

- **Porridge oats with milk, cinnamon, grated apple and 1 tablespoon milled flaxseed**
- **Natural yoghurt topped with sugar-free granola (page 148) and berries**
- **Supercharger smoothie (page 152)**
- **Poached egg(s) served with tomato and one slice of wholegrain toast**
- **1 power pancake (page 151)**
- **3 oatcakes topped with Edam or cottage cheese and sliced apple**
- **3 oatcakes topped with nut butter and sliced apple or pear**
- **3 oatcakes topped with hard-boiled egg and sliced tomato or cucumber**

• Lunch suggestions •

SOUPS

Soup is a comforting lunch option, particularly on cold winter days, and it's a great way to get your veggies in. Just make sure to always include a source of protein in your soup or on the side so that it's a balanced meal. If it's a filling soup with plenty of protein and veg, you may not need to have anything on the side. If you'd like something on the side, a couple of oatcakes or rye crispbreads with a topping of your choice is a great alternative to bread.

For convenience, consider making up a large batch of soup in advance that you can store in the fridge or freezer. Put some soup into a thermos flask or a transportable container to reheat in work.

EGGS

Eggs are a great lunch option because they're quick to make and versatile as well as filling. Omelettes are particularly flexible. You can eat them plain or with anything from one to a dozen ingredients, including onions, mushrooms, tomatoes, cheese, spinach, herbs or courgettes. See page 164 for my veggie omelette recipe.

SANDWICHES

So many people are stuck in a sandwich rut at lunchtime, which means they end up eating a lot of bread and miss out on other, more healthful lunch options.

Don't get into the habit of eating sandwiches or bread for lunch on a daily basis. If you do choose to have a sandwich, make sure to include a good portion of protein, such as tuna or chicken, and include plenty of salad. When choosing a bread, opt for a sugar-free variety with a minimum of 2 grams of fibre per slice, ideally more. Wholegrain bread is best. Look for bread made from either (or a combination of) wholegrain wheat, whole rye, whole oats, wheat germ, amaranth, barley, buckwheat, millet, spelt, quinoa or bulgur.

Moderation is key: two slices of bread in a day is more than enough, particularly if you're watching your weight.

SALADS

Choose a protein-rich food or a combination. Here are some ideas: chicken, turkey, ham, hard-boiled egg, hummus, mozzarella, feta, tuna, salmon, sardines, chickpeas, butter beans, kidney beans, cannellini beans. For convenience, tinned fish and beans are acceptable.

Combine the protein with a range of salads or veggies. Here are some ideas: mixed leaves, rocket, baby spinach, avocado, tomatoes, peppers, cucumbers, grated carrot or courgette, celery, onion, sprouts.

Add a healthy dressing (optional). A tablespoon of olive oil with a teaspoon of balsamic vinegar works a treat. See page 190 for simple dressing recipes.

Add one portion of slow-release carbohydrate to serve with or alongside your salad (optional). Here are some ideas: oatcakes, rye crispbread, wholegrain bread, quinoa, bulgur wheat, brown rice, wholemeal pasta.

LEFTOVERS

I'm a big fan of making lunch out of leftovers from last night's dinner. I often take this into consideration at dinnertime by cooking a little extra, or if I fancy a second helping at dinner, I console myself by deciding to have that second helping for lunch instead the following day. That way I get two meals out of what I've cooked and never feel too full.

TOP TIP

I OFTEN COOK UP A POT OF QUINOA AT THE START OF THE WEEK, STORE IT IN THE FRIDGE AND THEN ADD IT TO SOUPS AND SALADS AT LUNCHTIME. KEEPING A FEW COOKED HARD-BOILED EGGS IN THE FRIDGE IS ALSO SUPER HANDY FOR A QUICK BUT FILLING LUNCH OR SNACK.

Lunch ideas

- Chicken, vegetable and barley soup with a hint of ginger (page 157)
- Tuna salad sandwich on wholegrain bread
- 3 or 4 oatcakes or rye crispbreads topped with hummus (page 187), cheese or tuna with slices of tomato or cucumber on top
- Ham, coleslaw and hard-boiled egg salad
- Scrumptious veggie omelette (page 164)
- Simple 'n' smooth veggie lentil soup (page 156)
- Tomato, mozzarella and chickpea salad (page 161)
- Quinoa, avocado and tomato salad
- Bulgur salad with feta and blueberries (page 162)

Snack suggestions

- A palmful of **nuts or seeds** with a piece of fruit
- **Natural yoghurt** topped with stewed apple or fresh berries
- **1 or 2 oatcakes** topped with cheese, hummus (page 187), hard-boiled egg or nut butter
- **Raw veggie sticks with hummus** (page 187) – red pepper, celery and carrot work well
- **Almond butter** spread on sliced apple
- **Supercharger smoothie** (page 152)
- **Simple guacamole with crudités** (page 189)

Below are a few options if you fancy having an *occasional* sweet-ish treat. However, you should avoid consuming any of the sweet snack options until you have been on the Perfect Balance Eating Plan for *at least* two weeks. If you introduce sweet treats too early on or too often, you may reawaken your sweet tooth and reignite old habits.

Sweet-ish snack ideas

- A couple squares of good-quality dark chocolate (minimum 70% cocoa)
- 1 dark chocolate-covered rice cake
- Stewed fruit (apple, pear, rhubarb) flavoured with cinnamon or ginger and served with natural Greek yoghurt
- A small ripe banana or a small portion of dried fruit such as dates or figs
- Banana walnut bread (page 196)
- Health energy bars (page 199)

• Dinner •

As you've probably gathered by now, my approach to nutrition does not involve weighing food or counting calories or points, as I don't think that type of approach is sustainable for the long term. Instead, I simply encourage people to make healthy choices for themselves while following a few simple guidelines.

The important principles to remember when it comes to dinner are to use fresh, natural ingredients and, most importantly, to get the balance of nutrients right. As you know, a balanced meal should be made up of one-quarter protein (a serving about the size of your palm), one-quarter carbohydrate (e.g. 1 medium potato or 3 heaped tablespoons of rice) and the remaining half should consist of vegetables or salad.

What you choose to fill your plate with is up to you, and you can keep it as simple as you like.

Dinner ideas

- Chicken or pork stir-fry with garlic, onions, peppers, mushrooms and mangetout. Season with a dash of tamari or soy sauce and serve with wholegrain basmati rice.
- Baked salmon or cod served with sweet potato mash and asparagus
- Red lentil curry (page 168) served with wholegrain basmati rice
- A lean cut of steak served with baby potatoes and green beans
- Spaghetti Bolognese (page 182) served with whole wheat spaghetti and a large green salad
- Mediterranean chicken with roasted vegetables (page 180)
- Healthy shepherd's pie (page 178) with potato or cauliflower mash (page 186)
- Chicken and vegetable curry with wholegrain basmati rice
- Spinach, mushroom and tomato omelette
- Beef, mushroom and thyme casserole (page 176)
- Chickpea and quinoa burgers (page 170) served with rocket and cherry tomato salad
- Cheesy chicken and veggie bake (page 174)

• Beverages •

Aim to drink 2 litres of water per day. Avoid fruit juices, cordials, squash and soda, including diet soda and sugar-free soda, which contain artificial sweeteners (see page 116).

•

Next steps

NOW YOU KNOW almost everything you need to know in order to follow the Perfect Balance Eating Plan and live a low-sugar lifestyle with ease. The next chapter will further consolidate your knowledge by teaching you how to interpret food labels and recognise sugar substitutes. You'll also learn how to thoroughly enjoy eating out, socialising and going on holidays without going off track or feeling deprived.

What are you thinking?

Are you worried about whether you'll be able to sustain a low-sugar lifestyle in the long term? If so, reframe your thoughts into more positive, helpful ones. Here's an example.

Negative, unhelpful thought:

I'm not sure if I'll be able to keep this up in the long term.

Positive, helpful thought:

Thinking too far into the future is pointless and over-whelming. All I need to do is focus on what I can do today in order to look and feel my best *right now*. I can reassess things down the line if need be.

CHAPTER 7

GET SUGAR SAVVY

HOW TO
INTERPRET FOOD
LABELS AND
SEE THROUGH
MARKETING
JARGON

BEWARE
THE SUGAR
SUBSTITUTES

EATING
OUT AND
HOLIDAYS

How to interpret food labels and see through marketing jargon

TO KEEP TRACK of how much sugar – especially added sugar – you consume, you need to become somewhat of a sugar detective, at least in the early stages when you're educating yourself. This chapter will clue you in on what to look for on food labels, which is a valuable skill to have. Once you know what to look for, you can make better choices to limit your sugar intake and soon it will become second nature to you.

• Sugar in disguise •

Sugars appear on food labels under a variety of different names, so you need to know what to look out for. Two sneaky ways to disguise sugar on food labels is to use a long, scientific-sounding word or to rename the sugar altogether.

One of the easiest ways to recognise sugar on a food label is by the *–ose* suffix. When you find words that end in –ose, there's a good chance it's sugar, e.g. sucrose, fructose, glucose, maltose, dextrose, lactose (a naturally occurring milk sugar).

But just because it doesn't end in –ose doesn't mean it *isn't* sugar. For example, the ingredients list below for a low-fat breakfast cereal contains eight different types of sweeteners, and none of them end in –ose!

INGREDIENTS

Rice, whole wheat, **sugar,** whole oats, wheat bran, strawberry-flavoured apple pieces (dried apple, artificial flavours, citric acid, colour, sulphites), modified palm kernel oil, **corn syrup,** salt, **brown sugar syrup,** modified milk ingredients, **brown sugar, barley malt syrup,** rice flour, vegetable oil, polydextrose, monoglycerides, tapioca dextrin, shellac (confectioner's glaze), soy lecithin, yoghurt powder, maltodextrin, potassium sorbate, **honey,** modified corn starch, **blackstrap molasses,** cinnamon, **barley malt extract,** lactic acid, natural and artificial colours.

You'll be able to use your sugar-detecting skills to identify added sources of sugar in a food ingredients list such as the ones below. Although these substances are derived from a variety of sources, they can all be classed as some form of sugar.

You should avoid products that have one of these added sugars listed near the top of the ingredients list or contain several of them in smaller amounts. For example, the food label on the previous page would be one to avoid.

Terms to look out for on food labels:

Agave nectar

Barley malt

Beet sugar

Brown sugar

Cane crystals

Cane sugar or juice

Carob syrup

Corn sweetener

Corn syrup

Crystalline fructose

Date sugar or syrup

Dextrose, dextrin

Evaporated cane juice

Fructose

Fruit juice concentrates

Glucose syrup

Golden syrup

High-fructose corn syrup

Honey

Invert sugar

Maltodextrin

Malt syrup or extract

Maple syrup

Molasses

Raw sugar

Rice extract or syrup

Sorghum

Sucrose

Sugar, including granulated sugar, confectioner's sugar, turbinado sugar

Sugar alcohols, including sorbitol, xylitol, mannitol, maltitol (often found in mints and chewing gum)

Syrup, including brown rice syrup

• How do I know *how much* sugar is in a food? •

This is easy to figure out once you know how. On a food label, sugar comes under the heading of carbohydrates. Usually you will see something like 'carbohydrates 29g of which sugars 12g'. This tells us how much of the carbohydrate in the product comes from sugar.

Typical composition	100g contains	Per biscuit
Energy	1972kJ /469kcal	305kJ /73kcal
Protein	6.5g	1.0g
Carbohydrates	73.4g	11.3g
of which sugars	23.8g	4.0g

A simple and useful way of gauging sugar content is to remember that 1 teaspoon of sugar weighs 4 grams.

·1 TEASPOON SUGAR = 4 GRAMS

For example, if a granola bar contains 16 grams of sugar per serving, that's equivalent to approximately 4 teaspoons of sugar, which is a lot.

AS A GENERAL RULE, CHOOSE PRODUCTS WITH LESS THAN 5G OF SUGAR PER 100G OR 100ML.

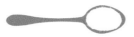

Less than 5g of sugar per 100g/ml = low sugar

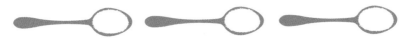

More than 15g of sugar per 100g/ml = high sugar

Dairy

Dairy is an exception to the rule above. Choose dairy products with less than 8g of sugar per 100g/ml. This is because with dairy, the first 4.7g of sugar per 100ml/grams listed will be lactose (naturally occurring milk sugars, which you don't need to be too worried about). Anything on top of that is *added sugar*, which we *are* concerned about.

For example, if you picked up a vanilla-flavoured yoghurt and it contained 15g of sugar per 100g, you'd know that only a third of the sugars present are naturally occurring sugars from the milk. The remainder is *added sugar*.

• Are ingredients listed in any particular order? •

You can also learn a lot just from looking at the order in which ingredients are listed. All ingredients must be listed in descending order by weight, including added water. The ingredient listed first is present in the largest amount and the ingredient listed last is present in the least amount.

This is an easy and quick way to judge a food. For example, if you buy an oat-based cereal, the first ingredient listed should be oats. Avoid foods where sugars are listed near the top or in a variety of different ways.

• Should I go by 'per 100g' or 'per portion'? •

Both are valuable in different ways. Nutrition labels will tell you how much of each nutrient is in a single serving of the food and in 100g of the food. Looking at the serving size information will tell you what you will get if you eat **one portion**, e.g. one 30g bowl of cereal.

The 'per 100g' part lets you **compare two foods that may have different serving sizes** (e.g. two different types of cereals) to see which has the most sugar per equal weight.

Watch out for foods that use small portion sizes on purpose. For example, many granola bars, which contain two parts, only count one part as a portion.

Don't be fooled into thinking 'low-fat' or 'diet foods' are the healthy choice. Here's why.

- When fat is removed from a food, it's often replaced with sugar and/or artificial sweeteners.

- Low-fat or diet foods often leave you hungry and craving more. One reason for this is that fat is filling and satisfying. For example, you are more likely to feel satisfied after one carton of full-fat yoghurt than one carton of low-fat yoghurt. In addition, fat slows down the release of sugars from foods, which keeps blood sugar levels from rising too rapidly.

- A diet low in essential fats can negatively impact on your mood, concentration, heart health, skin and reproductive system.

- People often think they can eat more of a diet food 'guilt free'. This can lead to overeating or bingeing.

• Keeping it real •

It's important to become more familiar with food labels, but it's equally important to remember that you only need to worry about them in relation to processed foods. Rather than obsess over the nutritional content between one food pack and another, you'd be better off sticking to natural whole foods as much as possible. That way, you know exactly what you're getting without having to fuss over food labels.

⚠ Beware the sugar substitutes

IT CAN BE tempting to reach for artificial sweeteners for a 'guilt-free' sugar hit. However, research suggests that artificial sweeteners can be just as harmful to our health, if not more so, as sugar.

I strongly recommend that you completely avoid all types of artificial sweeteners. These include aspartame, saccharine, sucralose and acesulfame k/acesulfame potassium.

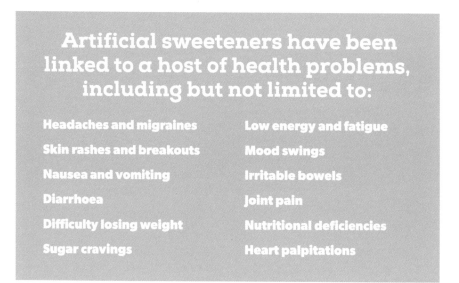

Artificial sweeteners have been linked to a host of health problems, including but not limited to:

Headaches and migraines	Low energy and fatigue
Skin rashes and breakouts	Mood swings
Nausea and vomiting	Irritable bowels
Diarrhoea	Joint pain
Difficulty losing weight	Nutritional deficiencies
Sugar cravings	Heart palpitations

• 'Healthy' sugar alternatives •

Now that more and more of us are becoming aware of just how harmful sugar and artificial sweeteners can be to our health, the hunt is on for 'healthy' or 'natural' sugar alternatives. Food manufacturers love to emblazon their products with 'natural sugar alternatives' to make them more appealing to consumers, but don't be fooled. Many seemingly natural substitutes aren't much better for us than real sugar.

I often get asked what the best alternatives to sugar are. Unfortunately, there is no simple, straightforward answer to this. I wish there was. There are many sugar alternatives on the market at the moment, but the reality is that research on the vast majority of them is still very limited and we haven't been consuming them for long enough to really know what the long-term effects might be.

For example, for the last couple of decades, agave nectar has been touted as a super-healthy natural alternative to sugar because it scores low on the glycemic index and therefore shouldn't spike your blood sugar levels. Health experts advised that it was great for diabetics and for anyone trying to reduce their sugar intake or lose weight. What's more, it looks and tastes almost identical to honey, so it seemed like the perfect alternative all round, right? Wrong.

Unfortunately, while on the one hand agave does have a lower glycemic rating than sugar and so it won't spike your blood sugar as quickly, there's a catch. Because on the other hand, we now know that commercial agave is a lot more processed than initially thought and contains more *concentrated fructose* than table sugar, most honey and even high-fructose corn syrup. Consuming high amounts of *concentrated fructose* can directly increase risk factors for obesity, heart disease and diabetes.

• But isn't fructose found in fruit? •

Yes it is, but that doesn't mean we should stop eating fruit. Allow me to explain, because there is an important distinction. The refining process in which agave nectar is made alters the chemical make-up of the fructose so that it becomes *concentrated*. *Concentrated fructose* is a man-made sugar. It is not found in fruit or anywhere else in nature. As a result, our bodies don't recognise it and we digest it differently than the natural fructose found in nature, i.e. fruit.

Fructose that is naturally occurring in whole fruits isn't isolated or concentrated. It's bound to other naturally occurring sugars and is accompanied by natural enzymes, vitamins, minerals, fibre and fruit pectin, which allow our bodies to digest and utilise it in a more healthful way. So while we should limit our intake of fructose, we shouldn't eliminate fruit from our diets.

And don't buy into the latest 'you can have any type of sugar as long as it's not fructose' craze either. *All* forms of sugar are detrimental to your heath if you consume too much of it, not just fructose.

I'm using the agave example to make the point that food manufacturers and health enthusiasts are constantly promoting 'the next big thing' when it comes to 'natural' sugar alternatives, but research into these so-called healthy alternatives is still evolving. What's 'healthy' one year will often be recategorised as 'unhealthy' the following year.

You'll always have people looking for loopholes – sneaky ways to have your cake and eat it too (pun intended). However, I (and possibly you) have been around long enough to have seen major diet trends come and go and to know better than to buy into the 'I can eat anything as long as it's organic/fructose-free/natural/paleo' or whatever the latest diet trend may be.

SUGAR IS SUGAR. NO MATTER WHAT THE SOURCE, IT CAN BE DETRIMENTAL TO YOUR HEALTH AND WEIGHT IF YOU CONSUME TOO MUCH. MY PERSONAL MOTTO IS:
'IF IT SEEMS TOO GOOD TO BE TRUE, IT PROBABLY IS. SO IF IN DOUBT, LEAVE IT OUT.'

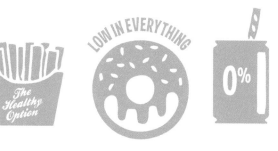

In addition, using sugar alternatives, no matter how natural they seem, is counter-productive when trying to reduce your sweet tooth and reset your taste buds. The bottom line is that if you continue to regularly eat sweet foods, you will always have a sweet tooth.

Once you have completed the 10-Day Sugar Challenge, you will notice a dramatic reduction in your desire for sweetness. As long as you continue to eat a low-sugar diet (as per the Perfect Balance Eating Plan), your taste buds will become more and more sensitive to sweetness, so you'll need less and less to feel satisfied. Through-out this book I've steered the meal ideas and recipes towards the less sweet end of the spectrum to help reset your palate towards less sweet foods.

Using sugar or sugar alternatives in *very small quantities* now and again isn't a problem, but if you use them regularly or in large amounts, it will hold you back and keep feeding your sweet tooth. The more highly refined a sweetener is, the worse it is for your body. If you want to add a little sweetness to your food now and again, I personally favour using fruit or the more naturally derived options in very small quantities, such as raw honey, maple syrup or perhaps green leaf stevia. Of these, current research suggests that green leaf stevia will have the least impact on your blood sugar. However, not enough people have been consuming it for long enough to know what the long-term health implications might be, so my advice is to proceed with caution.

•

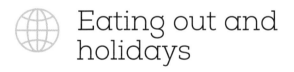

Eating out and holidays

YOU MAY BE wondering how your new way of eating will work when you're out and about and faced with limited options or unexpected food choices. I'm a big believer that dining out, socialising and holidays are to be enjoyed, and food plays a big part in that. There will always be occasions where you will have to adapt the Perfect Balance Eating Plan to work for you, and that's okay. Remember, this is a way of life, not a short-term 'diet'. Here are some tips on how to deal with social situations or holidays and how to cope with limited food choices when you're out and about.

• Eating out •

Once you get the hang of the Perfect Balance Eating Plan, eating out may be a lot easier than you think. As long as you balance your meal (¼ protein, ¼ carbs,

½ vegetables), you'll never go too far wrong when dining out. Of course, you may not always get the balance just right, and that's okay too. The aim is to do your best in any given situation.

The types of meals you want to avoid are those that are almost all pure carbohydrates, such as pizza, risotto, noodles or pure pasta dishes. For example, in an Italian restaurant you could order a chicken or steak and have some pasta as a side dish along with salad or veg. Or in a Thai or Chinese restaurant, rather than going for a noodle or rice-based dish, choose a dish that is rich in protein, such as meat, fish or tofu, and only have a small portion of rice along with plenty of veg. Sweet and sour dishes and Thai curries tend to be high in sugar, so they are best avoided.

Making smart choices will help you maintain a beneficial ratio of protein and carbohydrates, which will keep your blood sugar levels stable and leave you feeling full and satisfied. If you eat a high-carb meal, you'll be more likely to start craving chocolate or dessert afterwards.

• Tips for dining out at home or on holidays •

ALWAYS EAT A SMALL SNACK BEFORE YOU GO OUT

This will take the edge off your hunger and keep your glucose levels up. If you arrive at a venue starving and with low blood sugar, you'll be much more likely to start diving into the bread basket or make poor food choices. See the snack suggestions on page 107 for ideas.

DRINK ALCOHOL WITH FOOD

Having a couple of drinks before a meal will spike your blood sugar and increase your appetite, so you'll be more likely to overeat at dinner. It also means that the alcohol will likely go to your head, which will weaken your resolve for eating healthily. If you want to have a drink or two, I recommend you do so alongside your meal so that the alcohol is absorbed with the food. You'll be glad you did come the morning!

REVIEW THE MENU BEFOREHAND

Where possible, it may be a good idea to review the menu (online or otherwise) and decide what you're going to eat before you visit a restaurant. This is advisable in the early stages of following the Perfect Balance Eating Plan, when you are still learning how to adapt the plan to your lifestyle. Soon it will become second nature and won't require much thought or advance planning.

CHOOSE SAUCES WISELY

Watch out for hidden sugars in sauces, dips, pickles and condiments. If a sauce tastes sweet, it's likely to be high in sugar. If in doubt, leave it out or at least limit your consumption. Sauces to limit or avoid include ketchup, barbecue sauce, HP sauce, thousand island dressing, sweet chilli sauce, honey mustard, sweet tomato or pepper relish and onion marmalade.

KEEP IT SIMPLE

If you're unsure, the fallback in any restaurant is to choose something simple and ask for sauces on the side. For example, you can't go wrong with grilled meat, fish or chicken with salad or vegetables. Don't be afraid to ask for something that's not on the menu or have it cooked according to your taste. For instance, if you like the sound of fish cakes but don't like the sound of the sweet chilli sauce, ask for a different sauce or lemon or lime wedges instead.

AVOID DESSERT

It goes without saying that desserts in restaurants and cafés are loaded with sugar and therefore are best avoided altogether, particularly if you eat out often. Some people are capable of having a sweet treat on occasion and leaving it at that. Others who are particularly sensitive to sugar or prone to binge eating are not capable of having occasional sweet treats – it's all or nothing.

Deep down, you know which type you are. Be honest with yourself and experiment if you wish, but my advice is to err on the side of caution, particularly in the early stages. Why risk undoing all your good work? Remind yourself of what you have to gain by reading your benefits list (page 26) whenever you feel tempted.

No is good!

Remember, when you say 'no' you aren't depriving yourself – you're saying 'yes' to something better!

• On the go •

If you know that you're going to be away from home for the day and on the move with limited food choices, eat a filling breakfast such as eggs and pack a few healthy snack options like nuts, fruit and oatcakes to keep you going and away from unhealthy food options.

If your only option at lunch is to have a sandwich, opt for one with plenty of protein filling, such as chicken or tuna, and/or discard half the bread to make one generously filled sandwich. That way the ratio of carbs to protein is still favourable.

Of course, it won't be easy or even possible to stick to the plan all of the time, and that's okay. Plan ahead where possible, or if not, just make the best choice possible in your situation and get back on track with your next meal.

You'll learn as you go along how to prepare for, learn from and adapt to all types of food situations and make this plan work for you. In the next chapter, you'll learn how to overcome any feelings of deprivation that you may encounter down the line. But for now, be patient with yourself. I guarantee the results will be worth it.

What are you thinking?

Are you worried about your ability to handle eating out and socialising? If so, reframe any negative or unhelpful thoughts into more positive, helpful ones. Here's an example.

Negative, unhelpful thought:

Oh no, I won't have control over what I eat when I'm dining out or on holidays. What if I blow the whole thing?

Positive, helpful thought:

I'm following a flexible eating plan and the tips I've learned will allow me to enjoy eating out and socialising without problems. Over time, I'll learn how to prepare for and adapt to all types of food situations with ease.

CHAPTER 8

HOW TO AVOID COMMON PITFALLS:
THE KEY TO YOUR LONG-TERM SUCCESS

END MINDLESS EATING

NO MORE EXCUSES

BUT IT'S NOT FAIR!

FEND OFF FOOD PUSHERS

LET GO OF 'ALL OR NOTHING' THINKING

STAY ON TRACK

BELIEVE YOU CAN SUCCEED

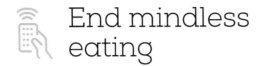

End mindless eating

DISCUSSIONS ON HEALTHY eating tend to focus on *what* we eat. Much less attention is paid to *how* we eat. Yet if you want to have a truly healthy relationship with food and manage your weight, you'll need to learn how to eat slowly and mindfully for the following reasons.

Firstly, when you eat slowly, your brain has time to register when you're full. Research shows that there is a time delay of up to 20 minutes between when your stomach fills up and your brain registers that you're full. The more slowly you eat, the more time you give your brain to register that you're full so that it can tell you to stop eating.

The second reason is that when you eat mindfully – and by that I mean when you pay attention to what and how much you're eating and savour each mouthful – you are much more likely to feel satisfied when the food is gone.

Mindless eating can be defined as eating food without paying adequate attention to what and how much is being eaten. Eating mindlessly undermines healthy eating and weight management by causing you to eat too much, make poor food choices and lose touch with feelings of hunger and fullness. You'll rarely feel satisfied after eating something mindlessly.

• Are you a mindless eater? •

Have you ever eaten a meal while watching TV or while working on your computer and then felt disappointed and dissatisfied when the food was gone? You may have thought, 'Where did it go? I feel like I've hardly eaten anything.' Or you may have looked down at an empty packet of biscuits and could hardly remember eating them. Or perhaps you eat on the run while completing various tasks or while getting from one place to the other.

If this sounds like you, I'd strongly suggest that you start engaging in some simple mindful eating practices, as set out on the next page. If you tune in to your body while you're eating, you'll enjoy your food so much more and will be more likely to feel full and satisfied with less food.

• How to become a mindful eater •

In the beginning you'll have to make a conscious effort to eat slowly and mindfully, but with practice, it will soon become second nature to you and you'll enjoy and digest your food all the better for it.

EAT SITTING DOWN

The best way to become more conscious of everything you put in your mouth is to only ever eat sitting down.

Most of the eating people do while standing up is impulse eating, like nibbling on something you see when opening the fridge to get something else out, grabbing a chocolate as you walk past an open box sitting on your colleague's desk or taking little bites as you prepare food or clean up after meals.

There's a real tendency to think that little nibbles here or there while going about your business don't actually count or won't have any consequences. But here's the thing: all the little nibbles here and there *do* count and *will* have consequences. It's important that you make every bite count.

Not only will eating sitting down make you feel more physically satisfied, it will also make you feel more psychologically satisfied if you see a full meal or snack spread out in front of you rather than grabbing bites here or there while on the move.

EAT SLOWLY

There are several reasons why it's important to eat slowly. As previously mentioned, the slower you eat, the more time you give your brain to register that you're full. In addition, eating slowly allows time for you to really notice and savour every mouthful and it enhances the digestive process.

To help you slow down, take note of the time at the beginning and end of a chosen meal. Once you have a rough idea of how long it takes you to eat a meal, you can work to prolong the time little by little at subsequent meals where possible.

A good way to train yourself to eat slower is to make a point of putting your utensils down a couple of times during the meal and taking a break from eating for a minute or two. Take a few deep breaths, have a sip of water or engage in some conversation before you resume eating. Take small bites and chew well.

PAY ATTENTION TO WHAT YOU'RE EATING

If you're distracted while you eat, it will reduce the degree of satisfaction you get from your food. Do what you can to eat in a relaxed environment. Where possible, turn off or move away from media devices such as the TV, laptops, tablets and smartphones. This way, you can focus intently on your food. Notice the flavour and texture of everything you eat and savour each bite.

HONE YOUR SKILLS

Try eating without distractions for one meal a day or even for a couple of meals a week to help you master the skill of eating slowly and paying attention to your food. Then incorporate these skills into your normal eating conditions as best you can. The idea is to minimise distractions when you eat, but ultimately you'll need to be able to eat slowly and mindfully even if you can't control your environment, such as when you're being distracted by your kids or colleagues.

'WHEN

WALKING, WALK.

WHEN

EATING, EAT.'

ZEN PROVERB

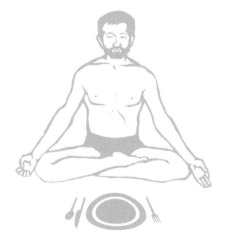

Eat slow = eat less

Several studies show that people do indeed eat less when they eat slowly. In one study conducted by nutritional scientists at the University of Rhode Island, researchers served lunch on two different occasions to 30 normal-weight women. The meal in both cases consisted of a plate of pasta with a tomato and vegetable sauce and Parmesan cheese.

At each visit, researchers instructed the women to eat to the point of comfortable fullness. However, during one visit they were instructed to eat as quickly as possible, while on the other visit participants were instructed to eat slowly and to put down their utensils in between bites.

When the researchers compared the difference in food consumption between the quickly eaten lunch and the slowly eaten lunch, here's what they found:

When eating quickly, the women consumed 646 calories in 9 minutes.

When eating slowly, the women consumed 579 calories in 29 minutes.

That is 67 fewer calories in 20 more minutes.

If you extrapolate that to three meals per day, you can see how quickly (pardon the pun) those extra calories could add up.

What's more is that when the women ate their lunch quickly, they reported more hunger an hour later than they did after their slowly eaten lunch.

So not only did eating quickly lead to greater calorie consumption, but it actually satisfied the women less. On the other hand, slow eating meant fewer calories but longer-lasting satisfaction, so it's a win-win all round.

No more excuses

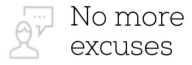

I'VE NOTICED THAT a lot of the weight loss clients I've counselled over the years have one thing in common: they're all very good at making excuses to justify their eating habits. While fooling others isn't ideal, fooling yourself is even worse. We all fool ourselves with excuses now and again (myself included), but how often are you doing it and is it hindering your progress?

• Who are you fooling? •

If you're in the habit of making excuses to justify eating something you shouldn't, then it's time you break this habit. Otherwise it will hold you back at some stage. The good news is that the solution lies entirely within your own control.

As with most bad habits, the first step to dealing with excuse-making is to acknowledge that you do it, and secondly to recognise *when* you're doing it. The tips below will help you do this.

• Recognise your excuses •

Excuses usually start with 'permission-giving thoughts'. Permission-giving thoughts are those little thoughts that whizz through our head giving us 'rational' reasons for things and helping us to justify what we're about to do.

These thoughts often start with the phrase:

'I PROBABLY SHOULDN'T

EAT THIS, BUT IT'S OKAY

BECAUSE...'

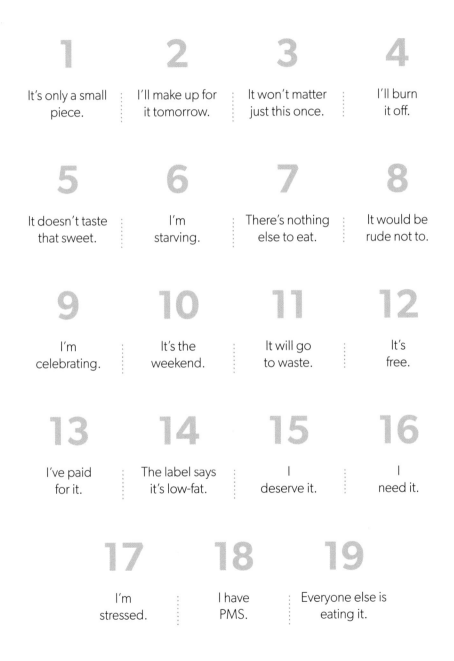

1 It's only a small piece.

2 I'll make up for it tomorrow.

3 It won't matter just this once.

4 I'll burn it off.

5 It doesn't taste that sweet.

6 I'm starving.

7 There's nothing else to eat.

8 It would be rude not to.

9 I'm celebrating.

10 It's the weekend.

11 It will go to waste.

12 It's free.

13 I've paid for it.

14 The label says it's low-fat.

15 I deserve it.

16 I need it.

17 I'm stressed.

18 I have PMS.

19 Everyone else is eating it.

We can allow other people to grant us permission too:

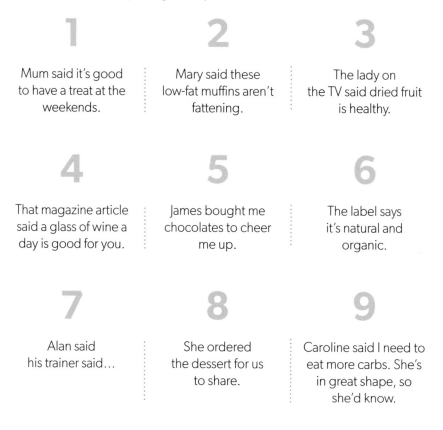

1

Mum said it's good to have a treat at the weekends.

2

Mary said these low-fat muffins aren't fattening.

3

The lady on the TV said dried fruit is healthy.

4

That magazine article said a glass of wine a day is good for you.

5

James bought me chocolates to cheer me up.

6

The label says it's natural and organic.

7

Alan said his trainer said…

8

She ordered the dessert for us to share.

9

Caroline said I need to eat more carbs. She's in great shape, so she'd know.

• How to stop making excuses and get your power back •

WRITE 'EM DOWN

Do any of those thoughts or excuses sound familiar to you? If so, write down the ones you've used in the past and/or are likely to use in the future. Seeing an excuse in writing helps you see it for exactly what it is. It also gives you the chance to reflect on and challenge your excuses while in a rational state, as opposed to when you're in the craving moment and in an irrational state.

The next time an excuse from your list pops into your head, part of your rational brain will recognise it for what it is even if you're craving at the time and having irrational thoughts. As the saying goes, forewarned is forearmed.

CHALLENGE YOUR EXCUSES

As you become more aware of the types of excuses you make, you'll be in a better position to challenge them.

When we're in the moment of really wanting to eat something, we often don't think with our heads and use *rational reasoning*, and instead we allow our stomachs and our emotions to do the reasoning for us. For example, convincing yourself that it's okay to have a chocolate croissant for breakfast because it's Sunday is not using rational reasoning.

Think of a common excuse you use to eat something you shouldn't and challenge it now by asking yourself the following questions:

1	2	3
Is my reasoning for eating this rational?	Am I thinking with my stomach or my emotions?	Would that excuse stand up in court or would it be dismissed as circumstantial?

4	5	6
Has this rationale served me well in the past?	Will eating this help me reach my goal and desired outcome?	Can I think of a more helpful or reasonable alternative?

It can also be useful to come up with some helpful responses to your own excuses. Write them down and refer to them when temptation strikes. There's an example on the next page.

Challenge your excuses

EXCUSE

HELPFUL RESPONSE

IT WON'T MATTER JUST THIS ONE ONCE.

JUST THIS ONCE WILL LEAD TO ANOTHER AND THEN ANOTHER. EVERY TIME I GIVE IN, I REINFORCE BAD HABITS. EVERY TIME I RESIST, I REINFORCE GOOD HABITS THAT WILL GET ME CLOSER TO MY GOAL.

I'VE HAD A TOUGH DAY. I NEED TO RELAX WITH A CUP OF TEA AND SOME BISCUITS.

I DO NEED TO RELAX, BUT I DON'T NEED BISCUITS. I CAN WATCH A MOVIE, READ MY BOOK, MEDITATE OR TAKE A BATH INSTEAD.

STAY ACCOUNTABLE

Another way we commonly fool ourselves is by underestimating or 'forgetting' how much we're actually eating in a day. You'd be surprised what our minds both naturally forget and conveniently forget when we don't really want to remember.

It's not that we're consciously trying to deceive ourselves about what we've eaten. It's just that it's really easy to forget about all the little nibbles or extra spoonfuls here or there and then we wonder why we're not getting the results we want. If this sounds like you, then I suggest that you keep a daily food and drink log to help you monitor your eating habits.

Writing down everything you eat and drink, including all the little extras you hadn't planned to eat, forces you to be aware of exactly what you're consuming and to be accountable for the consequences. It also helps you recognise and solve problems that may be hindering your progress. This is particularly relevant if weight loss is a goal for you. In fact, several studies show that keeping a written record of what you eat increases the likelihood that you'll lose weight and keep it off. Why not increase your chances of success in any way you can?

•

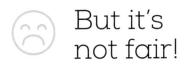

But it's not fair!

EMMA IS OUT with a group of girlfriends for dinner. Everyone is ordering dessert. Emma feels left out and starts to feel sorry for herself. She thinks, 'It's not fair that everyone else gets to have dessert except me' and starts to feel deprived and resentful. Then she thinks, 'Why should I be the odd one out? I deserve a treat too', and so she gives in and orders the sticky toffee pudding.

Like Emma, many people give themselves permission to eat something they oughtn't when confronted with feelings of unfairness. You might be one of them. I see many people fall into the 'it's not fair' trap and use the unfairness card as an excuse to deviate from their eating plan.

Can you relate to any of the thoughts on the next page?

IT'S UNFAIR THAT...

I CAN'T
ENJOY EATING AND
DRINKING WHATEVER
I FANCY WHEN
I'M OUT.

I CAN'T EAT
WHAT I WANT.
I CAN'T EAT LIKE
OTHER PEOPLE.

I'M NOT
NATURALLY SLIM
OR I HAVE A SLOW
METABOLISM.

I HAVE
TO DEPRIVE
MYSELF.

I HAVE TO
PUT SO MUCH EFFORT
INTO COOKING
AND PREPARING
FOODS.

Most of us struggle with the belief that life *should* be fair, but as you've probably gathered by now, life isn't fair. While we all have a certain amount of 'it's not fair' thoughts, how you *choose* to react to these thoughts is what really counts. Each choice has very different consequences.

You can either feel sorry for yourself, eat whatever you want, never look and feel your best, put your health at risk and continue to feel unhappy in yourself, or you can acknowledge and accept your feelings of unfairness for what they are, but still go ahead and do what you need to do, knowing that you'll be rewarded with looking and feeling your best.

Now that you've considered your options, do you think it's better to feel sorry for yourself and struggle with unfairness or accept it and take positive action? To help you make the best choice, do the following:

- **Read your benefits list on page 26** and remind yourself of all of the amazing benefits you'll get from eating healthily. Then ask yourself the following questions: 'Am I willing to let sugar prevent me from experiencing all of these wonderful benefits? Am I willing to let the "unfairness excuse" prevent me from reaching my health goals?'

- **Recognise that you're just feeling sorry for yourself** and put things into perspective by reminding yourself that everyone experiences some kind of unfairness in their life. This is just one of yours. Besides, are you really being deprived of something good?

- **Challenge your thoughts.** When you're feeling deprived, you may feel as though everyone around you gets to eat whatever they want. But that's simply not the case. I'm willing to bet that the vast majority of people *do* have to make sacrifices and eat in a healthful way in order to look and feel their best. I know I do. Why should you be any different?

What are you thinking?

Are you struggling with feelings of deprivation or unfairness? If so, reframe your thoughts into more positive, helpful ones. Here's an example.

Negative, unhelpful thought:
It's not fair that I can't eat 'normally' like everyone else.

Positive, helpful thought:
If I'm honest with myself, I probably wasn't eating 'normally' before I started this programme. I was eating too much junk food. I'm eating 'normally' now for a person who has a goal to be slim and healthy.

Fend off food pushers

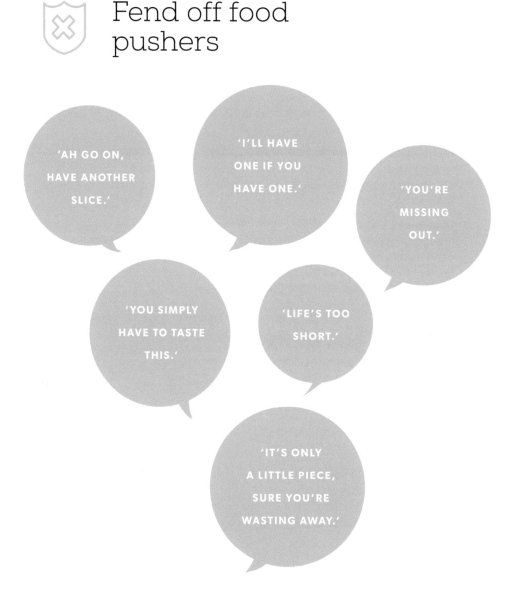

THERE IS ONE obstacle that almost every person trying to change their eating habits or lose weight encounters at some stage, and that's the food pusher. Food pushers are people who get a need within them fulfilled by getting you to eat.

They may only feel like a good host when others enjoy their food, or they don't like to eat or drink alone so they want you to join them, or perhaps they feel threatened by or jealous of your new lifestyle or appearance. Most of the time food pushing is unintentional and well-meaning, but whatever *their* motivation may be, food pushers can seriously sabotage *your* healthy eating plans – if you let them.

When you're offered a food that's not beneficial to you, the best response is a firm 'no, thank you' without any explanation, because excuses often open the door for opinions, arguments or persuasion. Don't feel the need to justify yourself.

However, some people won't be silenced easily and will try to persuade you for a variety of reasons. That's when it can be helpful to just be honest about what you're going through and ask them for their understanding and support. Bringing the issue out into the open in a non-defensive manner may be all that's needed. For example, it simply may not have occurred to your aunt that her fruitcake is not the best choice for someone who's watching their blood sugar. Perhaps she needs to be told.

If you find it difficult to say no to food pushers, it may be worth exploring *why* you feel this way. In my experience, it's usually for at least one of the following reasons:

1	2	3
Fear of offending, hurting or annoying someone by not eating what they want you to eat	Fear of drawing unwanted attention to yourself by not eating what everyone else is	Using either or both of the aforementioned as an excuse to eat something that deep down you know you really want to eat

• Fear of offending others •

Many clients tell me that they've found themselves in situations where they felt that they 'had' to eat something for fear of offending, hurting or annoying someone else. For example, Susan felt she couldn't say no to her mother-in-law's dessert at Sunday lunch, Sean felt he had to eat the buns his PA brought in on Fridays and Emma didn't want to draw attention to herself by not eating the birthday cake at her nephew's party.

Do you worry about offending others by not eating? If so, is it possible that you may be overestimating how much you'll offend someone by not eating? For example, think about how you would react if someone turned down food that you offered, particularly if you knew they were trying to improve their health or lose weight. How bad would you feel? How long would that feeling last? I think most people's disappointment would be fairly mild and fleeting. What do you think?

If you still find yourself assuming that others will be disappointed if you turn down food, ask yourself:

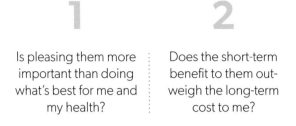

1

Is pleasing them more important than doing what's best for me and my health?

2

Does the short-term benefit to them outweigh the long-term cost to me?

It really is okay to disappoint others if you're dong it for the right reasons, especially when their disappointment is likely to be mild and fleeting. You're entitled to do what's right for you as long as you're polite in your refusal. Anyone who gives you a hard time is the one being unreasonable, not you.

• Fear of drawing attention to yourself •

Have you ever found yourself accepting unwanted food offers because it seemed easier to do so rather than risk drawing attention to yourself or being asked questions about your eating habits in front of others? Perhaps you can relate to Emma, who worried about what people might think or say if she didn't accept some cake at her nephew's birthday party.

These are all common and natural thoughts and behaviours, particularly if you feel sensitive about your weight and/or food choices. However, while it's perfectly okay to feel this way, it's not okay to let it sabotage your progress.

Fear of drawing attention to yourself often stems from fear of being judged by others. Do you find yourself worrying about what others think of you? Do you assume they'll judge you in a negative way? I know I've felt this way before.

In CBT terms, this unhelpful thinking habit is known as 'mind reading'. For example, when Emma thought, 'They'll think I'm weight obsessed if I don't eat the cake' or 'Kate will think I'm rude if I don't taste the cake she's made', this is an example of 'mind reading'. If, like me, you're prone to 'mind reading', you're probably aware that it can cause you a lot of unnecessary worry and anguish.

The trouble is that when we make assumptions about other people's opinion of us, we usually assume that it's negative. But the reality is that we have no way of knowing for certain what another person is thinking unless they choose to tell us.

Try to stop worrying what others think of you (even a little) and remind yourself that you only ever have control over what you think of yourself. It's a freeing thought. So why waste precious time and energy over something you have absolutely no control over?

'YOU WOULDN'T WORRY SO MUCH ABOUT WHAT OTHERS THINK OF YOU IF YOU REALISED HOW SELDOM THEY DO.' ELEANOR ROOSEVELT

Helpful responses to fend off food pushers

If you're offered something you'd rather not eat, choose phrases that acknowledge the person's feelings but still make your point: 'That looks amazing and I wish I had room, but I'm really enjoying the...'

If you're offered a second helping you don't need, keeping your reply in the past tense gives your words a sense of finality: 'It was delicious and I really enjoyed it, but I've had enough.'

THE PUSH: 'It's my specialty, you have to try it!'
YOUR RESPONSE: 'I will in a bit!'

THE PUSH: 'One bite isn't going to kill you.'
YOUR RESPONSE: 'I know, but once you pop, you can't stop! And I'm sure it's so yummy I wouldn't be able to stop.'

THE PUSH: 'But it's your favourite!'
YOUR RESPONSE: 'I know, but I think I've overdosed on it. I just can't eat it anymore!'

THE PUSH: 'We have so many leftovers, take some home with you!'
YOUR RESPONSE: 'Thanks for the offer, but I've a fridge full of food that needs to be used up. Just think, you'll have your meals for tomorrow taken care of.'

Let go of 'all or nothing' thinking

ONE OF THE most common traps I see people fall into is the 'all or nothing' syndrome. This is when you tell yourself you've blown it by eating one biscuit, so you may as well eat the whole packet. In CBT terms, this is called 'black and white' thinking – we have to be perfect or we're a failure; there is no middle ground. I find that this type of thinking is often used by those of us who are stuck in a dieting mindset, where you can only ever be on a diet or off a diet, with no in between.

However, real life is not that straightforward or clear cut. You will have days where you overeat or indulge in less healthy foods, and that's perfectly normal. You're human. It's okay to slip up now and again. What's not okay is allowing a small slip-up to turn into a big one and letting it derail you entirely. The example below illustrates this perfectly. See if you can relate.

Thoughts of a serial dieter: The 'all or nothing' syndrome

You're out for dinner on Saturday night and decide to have a few mouthfuls of your partner's tiramisu dessert. You really enjoyed the few mouthfuls, but shortly afterwards you felt guilty for eating it. After dinner you go to the cinema and decide that seeing as how you've already blown your diet, you may as well go the whole hog and get some ice cream. 'I'll get back on track tomorrow,' you tell yourself.

The next morning, you wake up feeling guilty about the previous night's indulgences and think, 'I can't believe I pigged out and completely ruined my diet. I've no willpower. I'm a disaster, I'll never be able to stay on this diet.' Feeling weak, ashamed and demotivated, you decide to have white toast with lashings of jam for breakfast. What's the point in trying?

However, by the afternoon you start to feel a bit better after a brisk walk in the park. You recall your weight loss goal and decide you need to get back on your diet. But then another thought creeps in: 'Seeing as how it's Sunday and

> I've already made a mess of the weekend, maybe I should wait till Monday to get back on my diet. I may as well just eat what I want for the rest of the day and start fresh tomorrow. After all, Monday is a better day to start. Hmm, maybe I'll pick up some chocolates for this evening since I don't restart my diet till tomorrow.'

I hope you can see that in the example above, enjoying a few mouthfuls of tiramisu wasn't the actual problem. It was the thoughts and actions that followed as a result that were the problem and caused the most damage. It illustrates how having a dieting mindset can lead to 'black and white' and 'all or nothing' thinking, which in turn leads to all sorts of problems.

REMEMBER, YOUR MINDSET CREATES THE FOUNDATION THAT INFLUENCES THE OUTCOME OF YOUR ACTIONS MORE THAN ANY OTHER VARIABLE.

The guidelines below will help you cultivate a balanced and helpful mindset that will keep you on track going forward.

• Lose the diet mentality •

If you're not 'on a diet', you can never 'blow your diet'. To foster a more positive mindset, practise saying, 'I am simply choosing to eat in a way that enables me to look and feel my best.'

• Focus on today •

If you focus on the past or the future with thoughts like 'I really blew it yesterday' or 'I'll never be able to keep this up', you'll feel overwhelmed and discouraged. That's why it's so important to view *each day* as an *individual opportunity* to do your best. What happened yesterday or what happens tomorrow is irrelevant. The most important action is what you're doing *right now*.

• Think progress, not perfection •

If you focus on perfection you'll probably view any slip-up as a total failure and start thinking, 'If I can't do it perfectly, then why even bother?' Does this sound like helpful thinking? Remind yourself that you're on a journey towards better health. You may go a little off course along the way, but each time you steer yourself back, you're making significant progress.

•

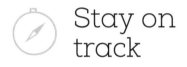

Stay on track

WE ALL GO a bit off course now and again for a variety of different reasons. This isn't a big problem *provided* you are able to get yourself back on track *sooner* rather than *later*. The quicker you get back on track, the easier it will be. Once you learn the essential skill of getting back on track *right now* (as opposed to tomorrow or Monday), you won't allow a small slip to turn into a big one ever again.

If you've gone off track and are struggling to get back on track, the following steps will help steer you back in the right direction.

1. Acknowledge and accept that you've gone off track.

2. Ask yourself which direction you want to go in. Any time you take a wrong turn on your health journey, you're left with two choices. You can keep walking backwards, which will take you further away from your goals, or you can accept your actions as human and forgivable and take not one, but two positive steps forward along the path that brings you closer to the future you want. To help you decide, read your benefits list on page 26 again.

3. Recommit yourself *right now*. Don't give yourself until tomorrow or Monday or January to get back on track. Draw a symbolic line, saying: 'Here's the line, right here, right now, where I stop this unhealthy eating.' Mark the end by taking some type of positive and relevant action, like going for a walk, making a healthy shopping list or reading your benefits list.

4. Give yourself credit for getting back on track and use the experi- ence as a learning opportunity so that you can lessen the chance of it happening again. For example, maybe you overate because you arrived to a party when you were too hungry or perhaps you neglected to stock up on healthy foods this week and so you ended up snacking on biscuits when you were hungry. You won't make the same mistakes again.

What are you thinking?

Are you struggling with 'all or nothing' thinking? If so, reframe any negative or unhelpful thoughts into more positive, helpful ones. Here's an example.

Negative, unhelpful thought:

Oh no, I've totally ruined everything by having that slice of cake. I may as well have another slice.

Positive, helpful thought:

Okay, so I shouldn't have eaten that cake, but it's not the end of the world and it won't undo the progress I've already made. I can start following my eating plan again right now. It's a hundred times better to stop now than to allow myself to eat more.

Remember, if you hit a rough patch at any point in the future for whatever reason, you can always come back to this book whenever you need to. You can reread the chapters and give yourself a fresh kick-start with the 10-Day Sugar Challenge if need be.

•

Believe you can succeed

CONGRATULATIONS! YOU ARE now well on your way towards living a low-sugar lifestyle and looking and feeling your absolute best. If you haven't already redone the Blood Sugar Balance and Wellness Assessment on page 32, I recommend that you do so after you've been following the Perfect Balance Eating Plan for around four weeks.

As you move forward on your journey towards better health, it's important that you continually take stock of all that you've learned and how much progress you've made since you started following this programme. This is so important because it will motivate you to make further progress and will build your confidence in your ability to do so.

Sometimes when you're doing really well at something, you're nearly afraid to believe it in case you jinx it or it ends somehow. You might believe your progress or results are a fluke or you just got lucky this time and you don't believe your progress will last. This kind of thinking often happens if, deep down, you don't truly *believe* you are capable of success, particularly lasting success. Self-doubt starts to creep in and cause sabotaging thoughts, such as 'I'll never be able to keep this up', particularly if you start thinking about past failures. You may be thinking, 'Why should this time be any different?'

But the good news is that this time *is* different! Here's a reminder why. Unlike before:

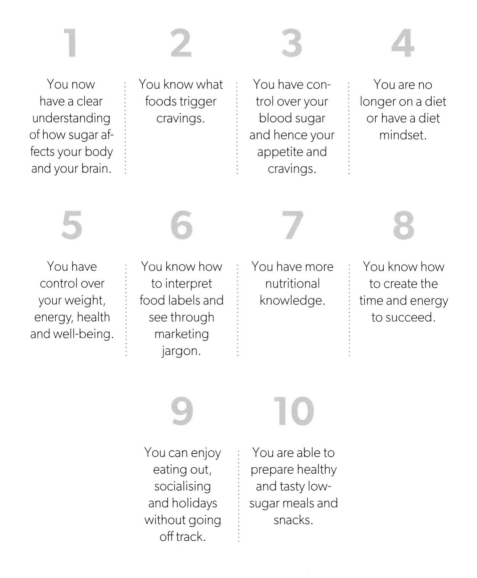

1 You now have a clear understanding of how sugar affects your body and your brain.

2 You know what foods trigger cravings.

3 You have control over your blood sugar and hence your appetite and cravings.

4 You are no longer on a diet or have a diet mindset.

5 You have control over your weight, energy, health and well-being.

6 You know how to interpret food labels and see through marketing jargon.

7 You have more nutritional knowledge.

8 You know how to create the time and energy to succeed.

9 You can enjoy eating out, socialising and holidays without going off track.

10 You are able to prepare healthy and tasty low-sugar meals and snacks.

And unlike before, you now have the mental and emotional skills you need to:

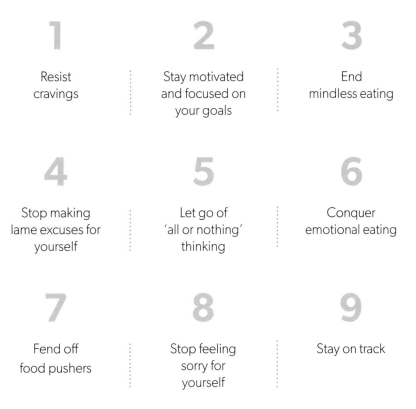

1	2	3
Resist cravings	Stay motivated and focused on your goals	End mindless eating

4	5	6
Stop making lame excuses for yourself	Let go of 'all or nothing' thinking	Conquer emotional eating

7	8	9
Fend off food pushers	Stop feeling sorry for yourself	Stay on track

If you can't fully believe in yourself just yet, that's okay, but at least believe in what you've learned.

You may not have total confidence in your ability to do all of the above right now, and that's normal. With time and practice, you'll get better and better at using these new thinking skills and you'll develop more and more confidence in your ability to do so. As clichéd as it sounds, practice makes perfect. Your progress won't disappear as long as you continue to use these tools.

Similarly, your new eating habits will become automatic for you in time. Be patient with yourself, learn from your mistakes and allow yourself the time and space you need to get to where you want to be. Remember, this is a journey, not a race.

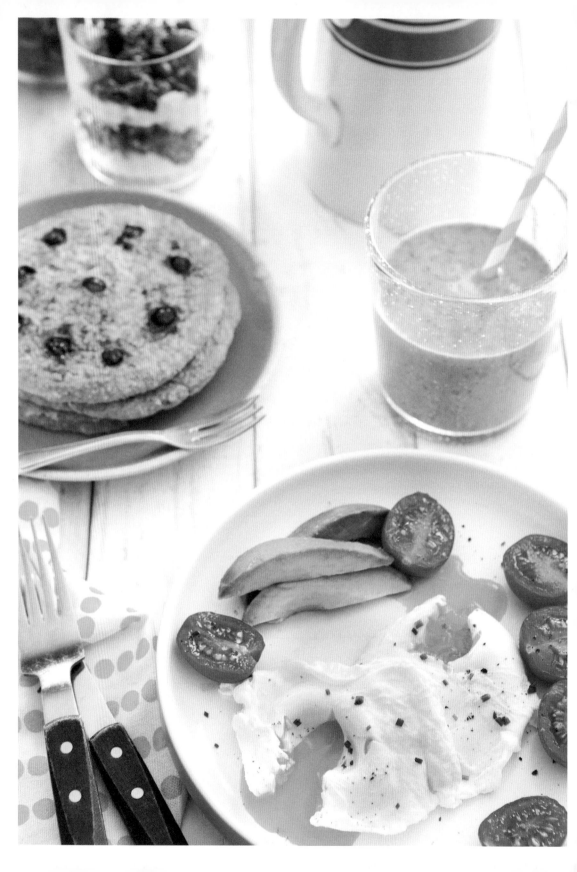

RECIPES
BREAKFAST

 = Suitable for the 10-Day Sugar Challenge

Genuinely Sugar-Free Granola

10

¼ cup coconut oil
1 cup oats
1 cup sunflower seeds
1 cup pumpkin seeds
1 cup chopped almonds (you can chop them in a food processor or use a knife)
½ cup ground flaxseed
2 teaspoons ground cinnamon
1 teaspoon almond extract or vanilla extract (I use both)
pinch of sea salt

Makes approx. 12 servings

It is virtually impossible to find a tasty granola that is genuinely sugar free. Most brands you'll find on supermarket shelves contain the equivalent of 3 teaspoons of sugar per serving, which is a lot. Even a lot of seemingly 'healthy' granola recipes contain lots of sugar in the form of dried fruit, honey or sugar substitutes.

The protein, fibre and essential fats in this granola will stave off sugar cravings and supercharge your energy levels at any time of the day. It works really well paired with natural yoghurt and fresh berries for breakfast or as a comforting snack to help ward off an afternoon slump.

1 Preheat the oven to 190°C. Line two baking trays with baking paper or grease lightly with coconut oil.
2 Melt the coconut oil in a small saucepan and set aside.
3 Place all of the remaining ingredients in a large bowl and mix together. Make a well in the middle and add the melted coconut oil. Mix thoroughly until everything is lightly coated with the oil.
4 Divide the granola evenly between the two trays and spread out in a thin layer. Bake in the oven for about 15 minutes, until lightly toasted and golden. Stir halfway through to avoid burning.
5 Allow to cool, then store in an airtight container for up to 1 month.
6 Serve with milk or natural yoghurt. It's also delicious served with fresh berries, grated apple or sliced pear.

Tip: Take care not to overcook as these ingredients burn easily and will taste bitter if cooked too long. I find that the baking tray that's placed on the lower shelf of the oven cooks a little quicker than the one on the upper shelf, so I take it out a couple of minutes earlier. You might need to do the same.

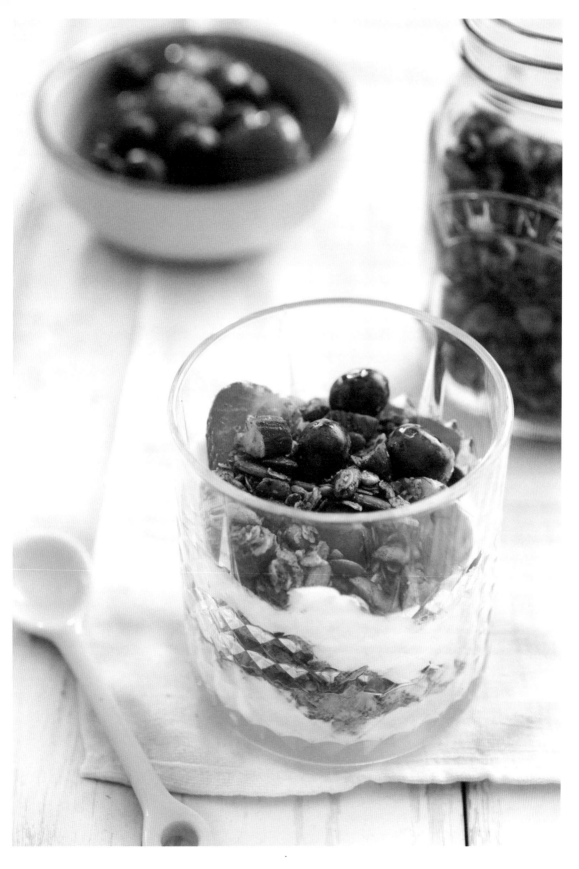

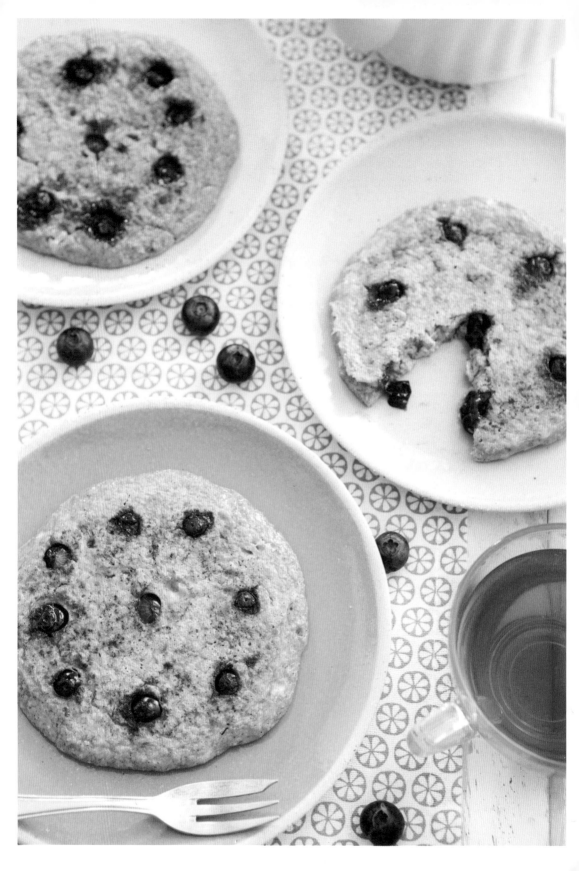

Power Pancakes

I call these power pancakes because unlike regular pancakes, they're high in protein and fibre so they'll keep you full and energised all morning. My toddler loves these pancakes as much as I do – not that he needs any help in the energy department!

100g cottage cheese
50g (½ cup) rolled oats
2 eggs
½ teaspoon ground cinnamon
small knob of butter or oil
handful of blueberries
natural Greek yoghurt, to serve

Makes 2 pancakes

1 Blend the cottage cheese, oats, eggs and cinnamon in a food processor or with a hand blender.
2 Put a non-stick pan over a medium heat and lightly grease with oil or butter. Pour in half the mixture to make one pancake.
3 Press in some blueberries all around the pancake and cook for 4–5 minutes on each side, until lightly golden.
4 Serve on its own or top with natural Greek yoghurt and extra berries.

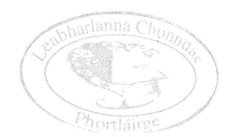

Supercharger Smoothie

1 ½ cups fresh or frozen
berries (strawberries and
blueberries work well)
1 cup unsweetened almond
milk
1 heaped tablespoon oats
1 tablespoon almond butter
1 heaped tablespoon shelled
hemp seeds or milled
seed mix

Serves 1

This smoothie recipe won't spike your blood sugar because it uses low-GI fruit and gives you a good dose of protein, fibre and essential fats that will supercharge your energy levels.

1 Combine the berries, almond milk and oats in a blender and blend until smooth. Add the almond butter and seeds and blend for another 5–10 seconds. Pour into a glass or travel mug and enjoy.

Apple and Cinnamon Bircher Muesli

10

Cooked porridge isn't the only way to eat oats. Oats eaten raw with cold milk are delicious too, particularly in summer. Bircher muesli is a traditional Swiss recipe that involves soaking the oats overnight, which really speeds things up at breakfast time. This is my version using oats, nuts, cinnamon, apple and yoghurt. I serve this in a ramekin dish, which makes me feel like I'm giving myself a little treat in the morning. It's the simple things in life!

1 Combine the oats, yoghurt, milk, cinnamon and vanilla extract in a bowl. Add the grated apple and mix well. Cover the bowl with plastic wrap or foil and leave in the fridge overnight.
2 In the morning, stir through half of the chopped nuts then scatter the remaining nuts on top of the oats. Top with blueberries or a fruit of your choice.

⅓ cup rolled oats
⅓ cup natural whole milk yoghurt
¼ cup milk of your choice (cow's milk or almond milk work well)
½ teaspoon ground cinnamon
½ teaspoon vanilla extract
½ apple, grated
2 tablespoons chopped nuts or a nut/seed mix (I use almonds and walnuts)
a few blueberries or other fruit, to serve

Serves 1

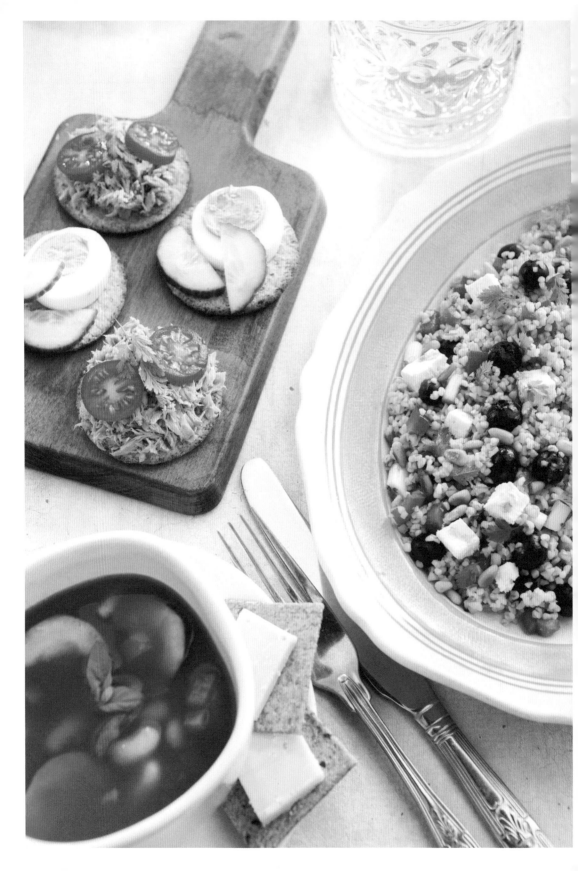

LUNCH

Simple 'n' Smooth Veggie Lentil Soup

2 tablespoons oil of your
choice

1 white onion, finely
chopped

2 garlic cloves, minced

1 teaspoon ground cumin

2 celery sticks, chopped

1 carrot, sliced

1 potato, peeled and diced

1 ¼ cups (250g) red lentils

850ml chicken or vegetable
stock

juice of ½ small lemon

fresh parsley or coriander, to
garnish (optional)

Serves 6

If you're not used to eating lentils, this soup is a great way to start, as the ingredients are so well blended you'll barely know you're eating them. I love this soup, especially in winter. I like knowing I can give myself and my family a bowl of goodness, particularly in the cold and flu season.

1 Heat the oil in a large pot over a medium heat. Fry the onion for a few minutes, until softened. Stir in the garlic and cumin followed by the celery, carrot and potato and cook for 5 minutes. Stir in the lentils and stock.

2 Cover and cook over a medium-low heat for approximately 45 minutes, until the lentils and vegetables are soft and tender. Remove from the heat and add the lemon juice.

3 Blend until smooth with a hand-held blender or in a food processor. Serve piping hot and garnish with chopped parsley or coriander.

Chicken, Vegetable and Barley Soup with a Hint of Ginger

Enjoy a bowl of goodness with this wonderfully comforting, aromatic soup. It's a nutritionally balanced meal in a bowl that will keep you full and satisfied for hours.

1 In a large, heavy pot, heat the oil over a medium-high heat. Add the carrots and leek and cook for about 7 minutes, until just tender. Add the diced chicken and the ginger and cook, stirring, until the chicken is opaque at the edges, about 3 minutes.

2 Add the stock and thyme and bring to the boil. Stir in the barley, then reduce the heat to medium-low and cover. Simmer for 25–30 minutes, until the barely is tender and the chicken is cooked through.

3 Stir in the spinach and cook for a minute or so, until wilted. Season to taste with salt and pepper and serve piping hot.

4 Cooled soup can be kept in the fridge for up to three days.

1 tablespoon olive oil
2 large carrots, quartered and then finely sliced
1 medium leek, quartered and then finely sliced
2 large or 3 medium chicken breasts, cut into 1.5cm pieces
1 teaspoon grated fresh ginger or ginger paste
1.4 litres chicken stock
4 sprigs fresh thyme
²/₃ cup barley
150g baby spinach
salt and freshly ground black pepper

Serves 4–6

Mediterranean White Bean and Vegetable Soup

2 tablespoons olive oil

1 medium onion, diced

1 courgette, quartered then sliced

1 red or yellow pepper, finely chopped

1 large garlic clove, crushed

1 level teaspoon paprika (I use smoked paprika)

1 x 400g can chopped tomatoes

juice of ½ lemon or lime

750ml vegetable or chicken stock

1 x 400g can cannel-lini beans, rinsed and drained

a few sprigs of fresh basil or 1 teaspoon dried basil

freshly ground black pepper

Serves 4–6

I love the combination of colours and flavours in this antioxidant-rich soup. It's as pleasing on the eye as it is on the palate.

1 Heat the olive oil in a large saucepan over a medium heat. Add the onion, courgette, pepper and garlic and cook gently until the vegetables begin to soften. Stir in the paprika, then pour in the tomatoes and lemon or lime juice. Simmer for about 5 minutes.

2 Add the stock and cook at a gentle simmer for about 15 minutes, until the vegetables are cooked but not soggy. Stir in the beans and heat for a few minutes more. Add in the basil and some freshly ground pepper.

3 Serve piping hot or cool and refrigerate or freeze until needed.

Variations

You could add a cup of cooked quinoa at the same time as the beans to make a more filling meal out of this soup.

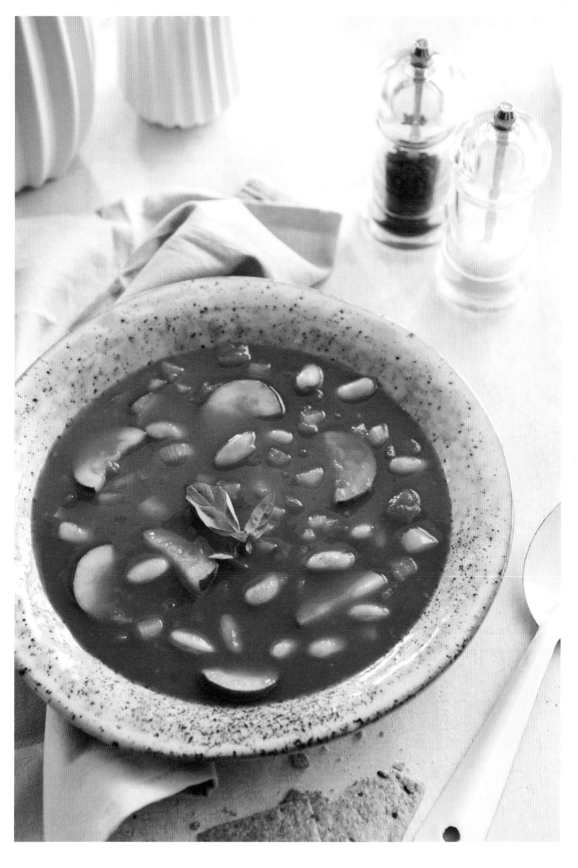

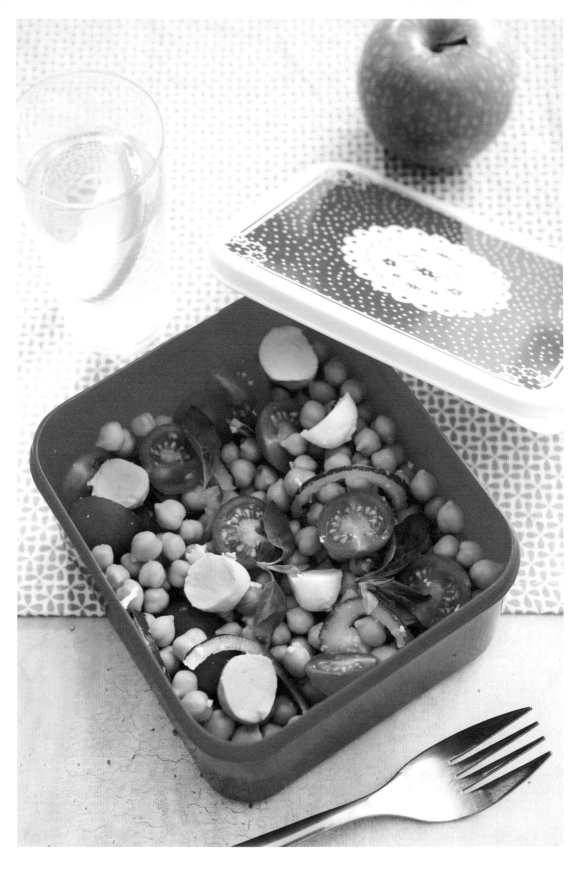

Tomato, Mozzarella and Chickpea Salad

10

Who needs sandwiches when you can whip up a tasty and filling salad like this in a matter of minutes? This is a really handy one to throw together in the mornings and it will hold well until lunchtime. Serve on its own for a satisfying lunch or as a side dish alongside a fillet of chicken or tuna.

1   Place the mozzarella, tomatoes, chickpeas and basil into a large bowl and season with a pinch of salt.
2   Mix the olive oil, lemon juice and crushed garlic together in a cup. Spoon over and mix through the salad ingredients.

125g mozzarella ball, cubed
1 cup cherry tomatoes, halved
1 cup tinned chickpeas, rinsed and drained
1 tablespoon shredded fresh basil
pinch of sea salt

DRESSING:
2 tablespoons extra virgin olive oil
1 tablespoon fresh lemon juice
1 garlic clove, crushed

OPTIONAL EXTRA SALAD INGREDIENTS
Red onion or scallions
Cucumbers
Black pitted olives
Avocado

Serves 2–4

Bulgur Salad with Feta and Blueberries

½ cup bulgur wheat, uncooked (or 1 cup cooked bulgur wheat)
1 cup freshly boiled water
pinch of salt
100g Greek feta cheese, chopped into cubes
4 scallions, finely chopped
½ red pepper, finely chopped
1 cup blueberries
¼ cup fresh parsley, chopped
¼ cup pine nuts

DRESSING:
2 tablespoons extra virgin olive oil
2 tablespoons balsamic vinegar
2 tablespoons fresh lime juice

Serves 4–6

This is one of my favourite summer salads. I love the combination of feta and pine nuts. The blueberries along with the balsamic and lime dressing add a touch of zingy sweetness that works surprisingly well.

1 Bulgur wheat does not involve cooking per se. All you need to do is place ½ cup bulgur wheat into a bowl or pot. Add 1 full cup freshly boiled water and a pinch of salt. Cover and let it sit for 20 minutes, until all the water has been absorbed, then fluff up with a fork. Allow to cool fully, then place in a large salad bowl.

2 Add the feta, scallions, red pepper, blueberries and parsley to the salad bowl and mix through.

3 To make the dressing, simply place the oil, vinegar and lime juice in a cup and give it a stir. Spoon over the salad and mix through. Sprinkle with the pine nuts.

4 Serve immediately or refrigerate until required.

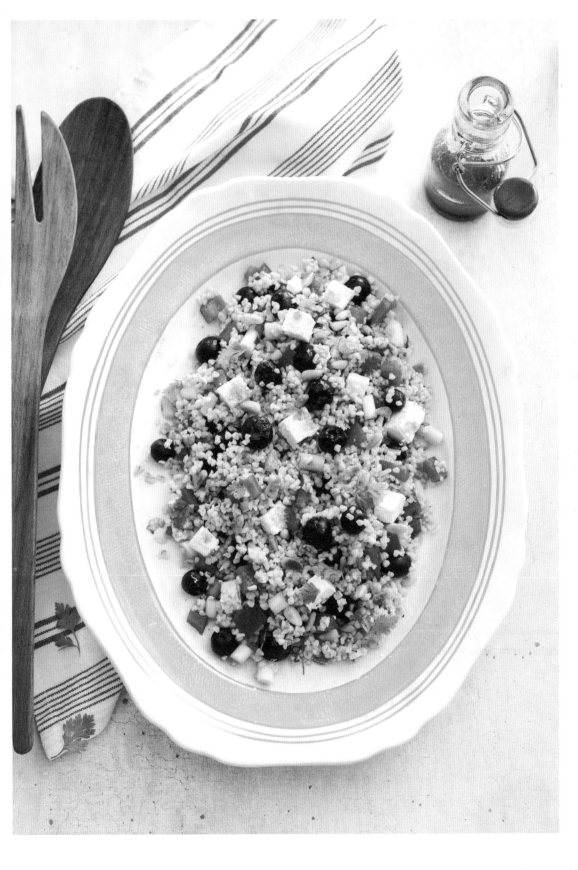

Scrumptious Veggie Omelette

1 teaspoon oil of your choice
½ cup sliced mushrooms
2 tablespoons chopped red
    pepper
1 tablespoon chopped onion
fistful of baby spinach leaves
2 eggs, beaten (preferably
    free-range)
1 tablespoon water
pinch of sea salt and freshly
    ground black pepper
1 heaped tablespoon grated
    white Cheddar cheese
    (optional)

Serves 1

I find eggs so filling and satisfying and I always feel really good after eating them. An omelette makes for a delicious breakfast, lunch or dinner in no time and you can use as little or as many fillings as you like. This is my favourite omelette recipe.

1   Heat the oil in a non-stick pan over a medium-high heat. Add the mushrooms, peppers and onions and fry for a couple of minutes, until softened. Stir in the spinach and cook for a further minute or so, until the spinach has wilted. Transfer the vegetables into a small bowl.

2   In a medium bowl, beat the eggs, water and seasoning with a fork or whisk until well mixed. Reheat the same pan over a medium-high heat and pour the eggs into the pan. Allow to cook for a minute or so while sliding the pan back and forth rapidly over the heat. Let it stand over the heat for 10 seconds or so to lightly brown the bottom of the omelette.

3   Place the cooked vegetables over half of the omelette and top with the cheese. Using a spatula, fold the other half of the omelette over the vegetables. Leave to cook for a few seconds longer, then gently slide the omelette out of the pan onto a plate and serve immediately.

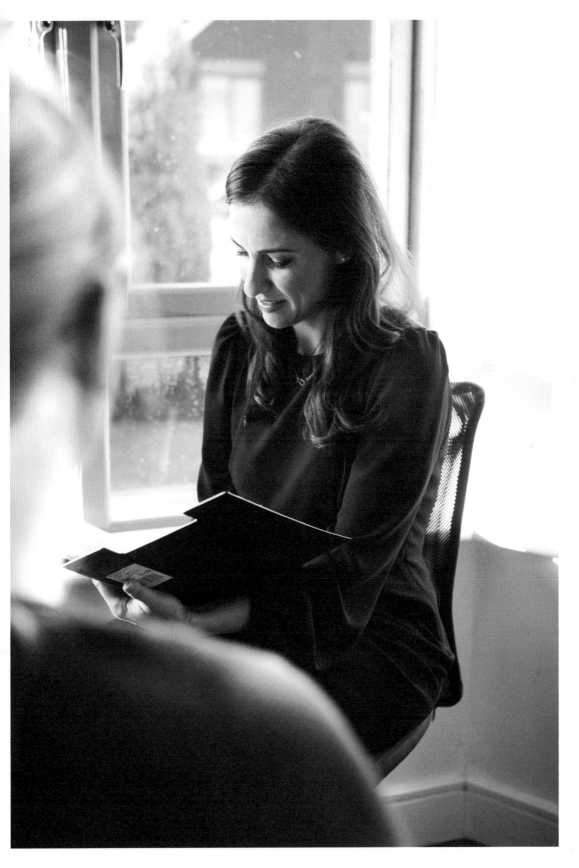

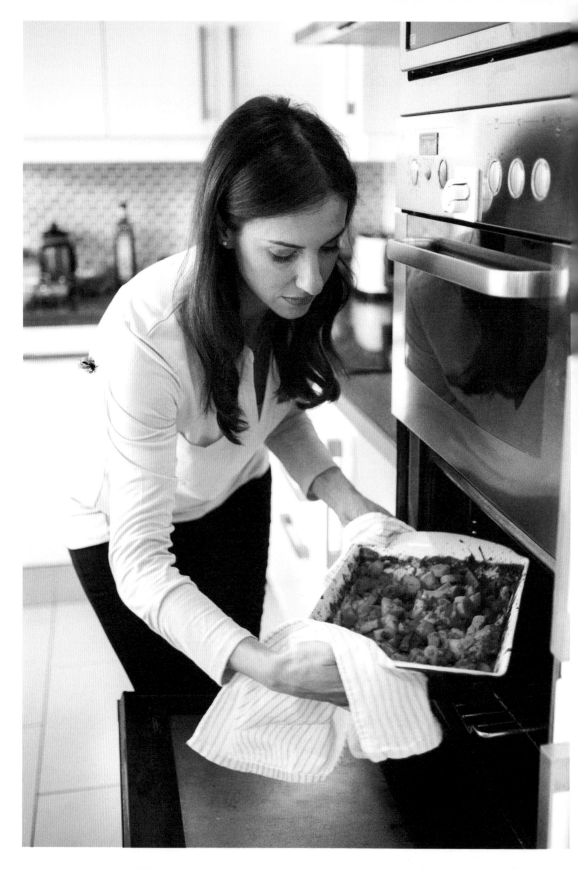

DINNER

Red Lentil Curry

2 tablespoons vegetable oil
1 large onion, finely
    chopped
2 garlic cloves, minced
1 heaped tablespoon finely
    chopped fresh ginger or
    ginger paste
2 teaspoons curry powder
1 teaspoon ground cumin
1 teaspoon ground turmeric
1 ¼ cups dried red split
    lentils
1 heaped tablespoon tomato
    purée
2 ½ cups water or low-salt
    vegetable stock
300ml coconut milk
juice of ½ lime
brown basmati rice, to serve
sprigs of fresh coriander, to
    garnish

Serves 6

This is a meal I really look forward to eating.
It took a while to get my husband round to
enjoying eating lentils for dinner, but this
recipe helped convert him. In fact, it's now
one of his favourite meals. Result!

1   Heat the oil in a large, heavy pot and fry
    the onion over a medium heat for a couple
    of minutes, until soft.
2   Add the garlic and ginger and cook,
    stirring, for 1 minute. Add the curry
    powder, cumin and turmeric and cook,
    stirring, for 1 minute more.
3   Stir in the lentils, tomato purée and
    water or stock. Cover and simmer over
    a medium heat for 15 minutes. Add the
    coconut milk and simmer for a further 15
    minutes, until the lentils are soft. Before
    serving, stir in the lime juice to add a hint
    of sweetness and bring out the flavours.
4   Serve on a small bed of brown basmati
    rice and garnish with sprigs of fresh
    coriander.

Variation
*Optional after you complete the 10-Day Sugar
Challenge – add 1 cup cubed butternut squash at
the same time as the coconut milk.*

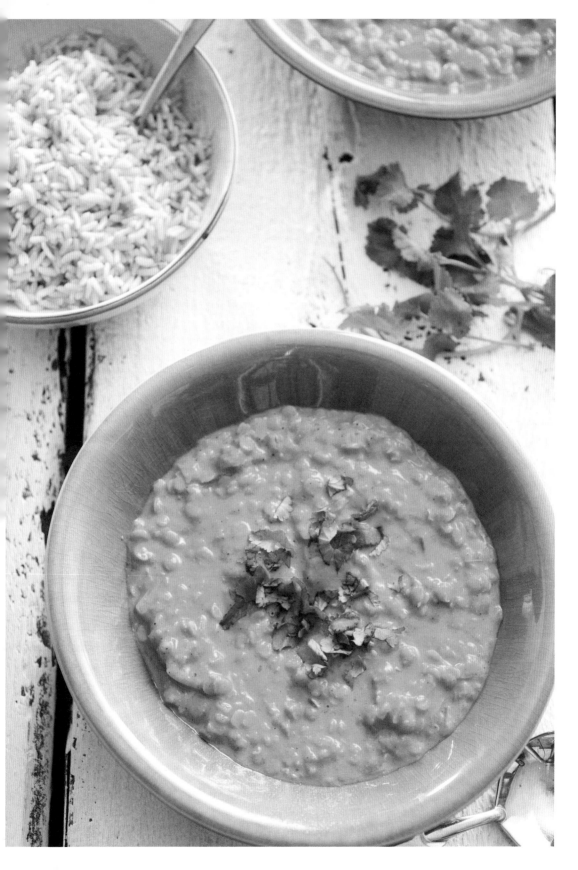

Chickpea and Quinoa Burgers

1 cup (approx. 200g) cooked chickpeas (if tinned, rinse and drain)
1 cup cooked and cooled quinoa
¼ cup rolled oats
1 egg
1 small red onion, finely chopped
½ red pepper, finely chopped
2 garlic cloves, finely chopped or minced
3 tablespoons fresh lime or lemon juice (I prefer lime)
1 tablespoon chopped fresh coriander
1 teaspoon sea salt
1 teaspoon chilli powder or paprika
1–2 tablespoons flour of your choice, for dusting
1 tablespoon oil of your choice for frying
green salad, to serve
guacamole (page 189) or salsa, to serve (optional)

Makes approx. 6 burgers

Many veggie burgers are dry and tasteless, but these ones are bursting with flavour. They're super quick to make, particularly if you use leftover quinoa. I love them paired with chunky guacamole or salsa and a crunchy green salad.

1 Place all the ingredients except the flour and oil into a food processor and pulse until well combined and fairly smooth.
2 Sprinkle some flour onto a chopping board as well as your hands. Scoop up some of the burger mixture and shape into the size of a golf ball, then press gently to make a burger shape. Continue until you have made six equal-sized burgers. Cover and refrigerate until needed.
3 When ready, heat a large pan over a medium heat and drizzle in the oil. Cook the burgers for about 4 minutes on each side, until light golden brown.
4 Serve with a green salad for a tasty and filling lunch or dinner. These also work well paired with guacamole or salsa.

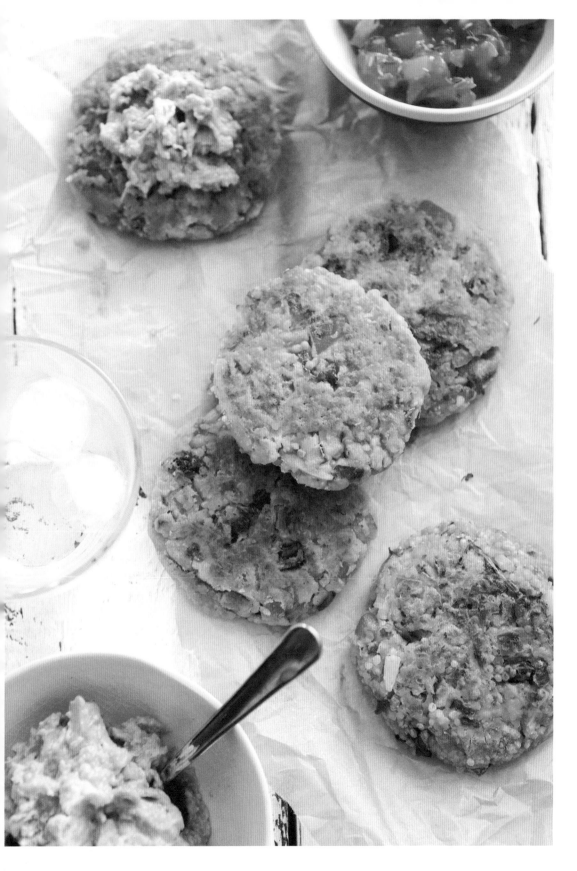

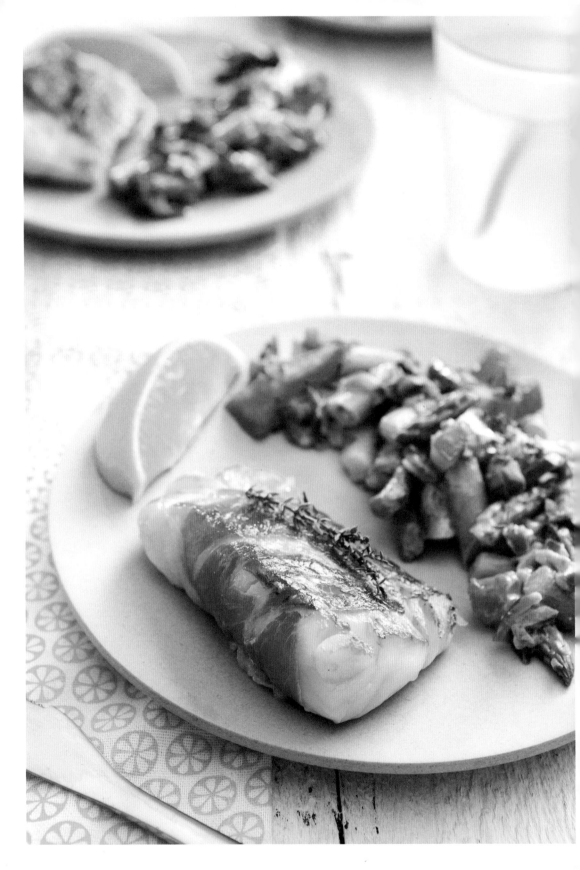

Prosciutto-Wrapped Cod with Warm Asparagus Salad

This meal is as nutritious as it is tasty. The cod is a good source of protein and the asparagus is a natural detoxifier. In fact, the entire salad is packed with antioxidant vitamins, which help to fight disease and make your skin glow. As a bonus, you won't have much washing up to do, as all that's required is a chopping board and a frying pan.

3 tablespoons olive oil

1 small red onion, finely chopped

1 teaspoon chopped fresh thyme

salt and freshly ground black pepper

2 teaspoons Dijon mustard

2 medium cod loins or skinned fillets

2 slices of prosciutto

200g asparagus, cut into bite-sized pieces

1 large, ripe vine tomato, finely chopped

lemon wedges, to serve

Serves 2

1   In a large non-stick pan, heat 2 table-spoons of the olive oil over a medium heat. Fry the red onion for about 7 minutes, until soft. Sprinkle over the thyme and season with salt and pepper. Stir through the Dijon mustard, then scrape the mixture into a bowl and set aside. Wipe out the pan.

2   Pat the cod fillets dry and wrap each one in a slice of prosciutto. Add the remaining 1 tablespoon of olive oil to the pan and set over a medium-high heat until the oil is rippling. Add the cod to the pan and fry for about 4 minutes on each side, until the prosciutto is crisp and the fish is firm and cooked through. Plate the fish and cover loosely with foil to keep warm.

3   Add ½ cup water to the same pan and bring to the boil over a high heat. Add the asparagus and cook for 3 minutes, then drain but leave in the pan. Add the onions back in along with the chopped tomato. Stir well and serve the warm salad alongside the fish with lemon wedges.

Cheesy Chicken and Veggie Bake

1 cup uncooked quinoa or 3 cups cooked quinoa
2 cups reduced-salt chicken stock
4 tablespoons extra virgin olive oil
½ teaspoon chilli flakes
½ teaspoon paprika
4 chicken breasts
3 cups broccoli florets
1 red onion, roughly chopped
1 x 400g can chopped tomatoes
1 ½ cups (200g) white Cheddar cheese, grated
¼ cup finely chopped fresh coriander or parsley
freshly ground black pepper

Serves 6

There's something very comforting about taking a golden and bubbling bake out of the oven of an evening. This dish is packed with quality protein and is a great way to use up leftover chicken and quinoa, which also speeds up the preparation time.

1 If you don't already have some pre-made, start by cooking the quinoa in the chicken stock according to the directions on page 188 and allow to cool. Transfer the cooled quinoa to a large bowl.

2 Preheat the oven to 190°C. Line a large baking tray with foil or parchment paper.

3 Put the olive oil into a cup and mix in the chilli flakes and paprika.

4 Arrange the chicken breasts on the baking tray and pour half of the oil and spices over the chicken so that it is evenly covered. Place the chicken in the oven and set your timer for 5 minutes.

5 Meanwhile, chop the onion and cut the broccoli into florets. When the buzzer sounds, add the broccoli and onion to the baking tray alongside the chicken and pour the rest of the oil and spices over them. Bake for a further 15 minutes. Allow to cool before you dice the chicken.

6 Add the diced chicken, broccoli and onion along with the oil and spices from the baking tray into the bowl with the quinoa. Add in the chopped tomatoes, half of the cheese and all of the coriander or parsley and season with black pepper. Use a spatula to combine the ingredients well, then transfer into a baking dish and top with the remaining cheese.

7 Cover with foil and bake in the oven for 15 minutes. Remove the foil and bake for another 10 minutes, until the cheese is melted and golden.

Note
You can also use leftover roast chicken for this dish instead of cooking the chicken breasts from scratch. About 1 cup of shredded roast chicken should suffice. If you do it this way, just bake the broccoli and onion alone in the oven for 15 minutes. You'll still use the oil and spices, but reduce the oil to 2 tablespoons instead.

Beef, Mushroom and Thyme Casserole

2 tablespoons oil of your choice

500g good-quality beef, cut into chunks (sirloin works well)

1 white onion, chopped

1 cup button mushrooms, halved

1 garlic clove, minced

2 teaspoons paprika (smoked paprika gives a delicious flavour)

2 medium white potatoes, peeled and cut into cubes

2 medium carrots, sliced

²/₃ cup frozen peas or petit pois

1 x 400g can chopped tomatoes

1 teaspoon fresh or dried thyme

200ml beef stock or bouillon

2 tablespoons crème fraîche (optional)

Serves 4–6

Highly nutritious and bursting with juices and flavour, this cosy casserole is a real crowd pleaser, particularly in the winter.

1   Preheat the oven to 165°C.

2   Heat 1 tablespoon of the oil in a frying pan over a medium-high heat and brown the beef in two batches. Lift out with a slotted spoon and put in a casserole dish as you go.

3   Wipe out the frying pan, then heat the remaining tablespoon of oil in the same pan and soften the onion over a medium-low heat. Add in the mushrooms, garlic and paprika and fry for a couple of minutes. Stir in the cubed potatoes, carrots, peas, tinned tomatoes and thyme, then pour in the stock. Add all the ingredients from the pan to the browned beef in the casserole dish and give it a gentle stir.

4   Cook for 1 hour 15 minutes, stirring occasionally, until the potatoes and carrot are cooked through. Allow to cool a little, then stir through the crème fraîche (if using) just before serving.

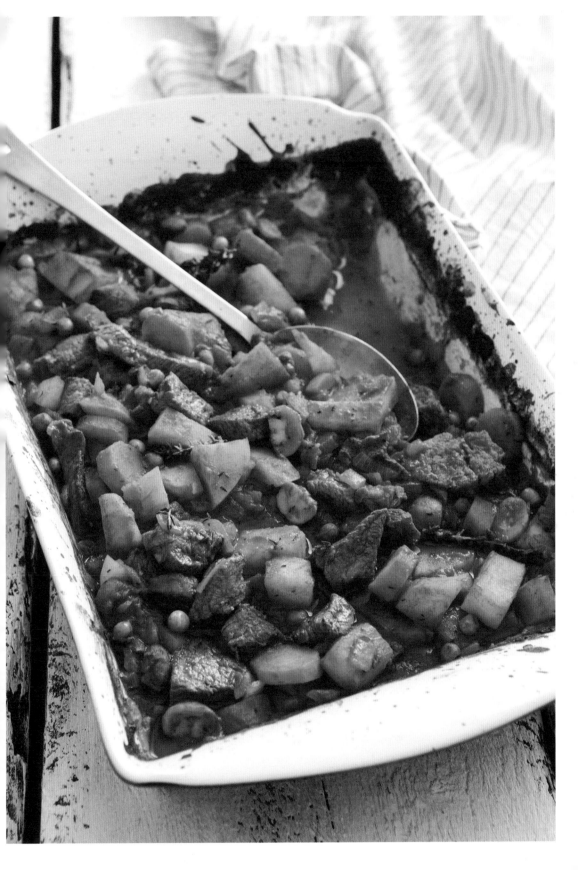

Healthy Shepherd's Pie

FOR THE FILLING:
1 tablespoon oil of your
    choice
1 onion, finely chopped
1 large or 2 medium carrots,
    finely diced
½ teaspoon fresh or dried
    thyme
250g lean minced beef
1 tablespoon plain flour
350ml vegetable stock (I use
    reduced-salt vegetable
    bouillon)
½ x 400g can chopped
    tomatoes
1 tablespoon tomato purée
1 teaspoon Worcestershire
    sauce
freshly ground black pepper
1 x 400g can green lentils,
    rinsed and drained

FOR THE TOPPING:
3 large potatoes, peeled
    and cut in half lengthwise
1 head of cauliflower, cut
    into florets
½ cup milk
1 tablespoon butter
salt and freshly ground
    black pepper

Serves 4–6

Tip: *This dish is suitable
for the 10-Day Sugar
Challenge if made with
the cauliflower mash
on page 186 instead of
potatoes.*

This is what I like to call 'healthy comfort food'. Substituting half the mince meat with lentils adds extra nutritional value and is a great way of slowly introducing lentils into your and your family's diet. Going half and half on the potato and cauliflower mash lowers the overall carbohydrate load of the meal, which is better for your waistline. And chances are no one will notice anyway.

1 To prepare the filling, heat the oil in a large saucepan over a medium heat. Tip in the onion and fry for 2–3 minutes, then add the carrots and thyme and fry for a further 5 minutes, stirring regularly.
2 Stir in the mince to break it up and fry for 2–3 minutes, until it's no longer pink. Add the flour and stir well, ensuring the meat doesn't stick to the bottom of the pan, and fry for a few more minutes. Pour in the stock and stir until thickened. Add the tomatoes, tomato purée and Worcestershire sauce and season with pepper.
3 Reduce the heat, cover and simmer for 20 minutes. Stir in the lentils, then transfer the mixture into an ovenproof casserole dish.
4 Meanwhile, to make the topping, bring the potatoes to a boil in a large pot of lightly salted water. At the same time, steam the cauliflower on top of the potatoes using a steaming basket or colander. Cook until both the potatoes and cauliflower are tender, which should take about 20 minutes.

5 Preheat the oven to 180°C.
6 Drain the potatoes and cauliflower and add them back to the pot. Stir through the milk and butter and mash well with a potato masher. Season with salt and pepper to taste.
7 Spread the mash on top of the meat and lentil mixture and bake in the preheated oven for about 20 minutes. Place under a hot grill for a few minutes at the end if you'd like to get a golden crisp on top.

Mediterranean Chicken with Roasted Vegetables

8 cherry tomatoes
4 large flat mushrooms, cut in half
1 large red onion, sliced into wedges
1 large yellow pepper, sliced into strips
1 courgette, halved and sliced into half moons
½ cup pitted black olives
4 tablespoons olive oil
3 tablespoons balsamic vinegar
3 garlic cloves, crushed
4 sprigs of fresh rosemary or ½ teaspoon dried rosemary
4 chicken breasts
salt and freshly ground black pepper

Serves 4

This simple chicken dish packed with Mediterranean goodness is my kind of food – colourful, flavoursome and nutritious. This dish can be served alone but it also works well served alongside quinoa, or you could roast thinly sliced baby potatoes alongside the vegetables.

1 Preheat the oven to 190°C.
2 Place all the prepared vegetables in a large bowl and set aside.
3 Pour the oil and vinegar into a cup and mix in the crushed garlic and rosemary. Pour two-thirds of the marinade over the vegetables and mix well.
4 Spread the vegetables across a baking tray. Nestle the chicken breasts on top and pour the remaining marinade over the chicken. Season with salt and pepper and bake in the oven for approx. 25 minutes, until the chicken is cooked through and the vegetables are nicely roasted.

Speedy Salmon Supper

Dinner is served in 10 minutes flat with this speedy number. Salmon is a wonderful source of omega-3 fats, which help to keep your heart healthy and support mental health and brain function.

1 teaspoon oil of your choice
2 skinless salmon fillets
salt and freshly ground
    black pepper
250g baby spinach leaves
2 tablespoons crème fraîche
2 tablespoons finely
    chopped flat-leaf parsley
1 teaspoon capers
juice of ½ lemon
lemon wedges, to serve

Serves 2

1 Heat the oil in a frying pan set over a medium-high heat. Season the salmon with salt and pepper, then fry for about 4 minutes on each side, until the flesh flakes easily. Leave to rest on a hot plate or in an oven set on a very low heat.

2 Tip the spinach leaves into the hot pan and season well, then cover and leave to wilt for a minute or so, stirring repeatedly. Spoon the spinach onto serving plates, then top with the salmon.

3 Gently heat the crème fraîche in the pan. Add the parsley, capers and lemon juice and season to taste. Spoon the sauce over the salmon and serve with lemon wedges.

Spaghetti Bolognese with Chunky Vegetables

2 tablespoons oil of your
   choice
500g lean beef mince
1 onion, chopped
1 large carrot, peeled,
   quartered lengthways
   and finely chopped
1 celery stalk, diced
1 medium courgette,
   quartered lengthways
   and cut into chunks
½ red pepper, finely
   chopped
1 cup button mushrooms
2 garlic cloves, minced
1 x 400g can chopped
   tomatoes
3 tablespoons tomato purée
250ml beef or vegetable
   stock
½ teaspoon dried oregano
2 teaspoons balsamic
   vinegar
salt and freshly ground
   black pepper
whole wheat spaghetti
   (amount depends on
   number of servings
   required)
handful of fresh basil leaves,
   chopped finely
freshly grated Parmesan
   cheese (optional)

Serves 6

Adding plenty of vegetables to your Bolognese sauce will help you achieve your 'five a day' target. It also bulks up your dinner plate, which allows you to use less pasta.

1 Heat 1 tablespoon of the oil in a large saucepan set over a medium heat. Add the mince, breaking it up with a wooden spoon, and cook until browned all over. Remove the mince from the pan with a slotted spoon and set aside.

2 Wipe out the pan and heat the remaining 1 tablespoon of oil. Add the onion and sauté for a few minutes. Add the carrot, celery, courgette, pepper, mushrooms and garlic and sauté for another 10 minutes, until soft.

3 Add the browned beef to the vegetables and stir in the tinned tomatoes, tomato purée, stock and oregano. Bring to a boil, then turn down the heat and simmer for about 30 minutes, until the sauce is thickened. Add the balsamic vinegar at the end along with salt and pepper to taste.

4 Serve mixed through a modest portion of whole wheat spaghetti. Top with chopped fresh basil and Parmesan cheese (if using).

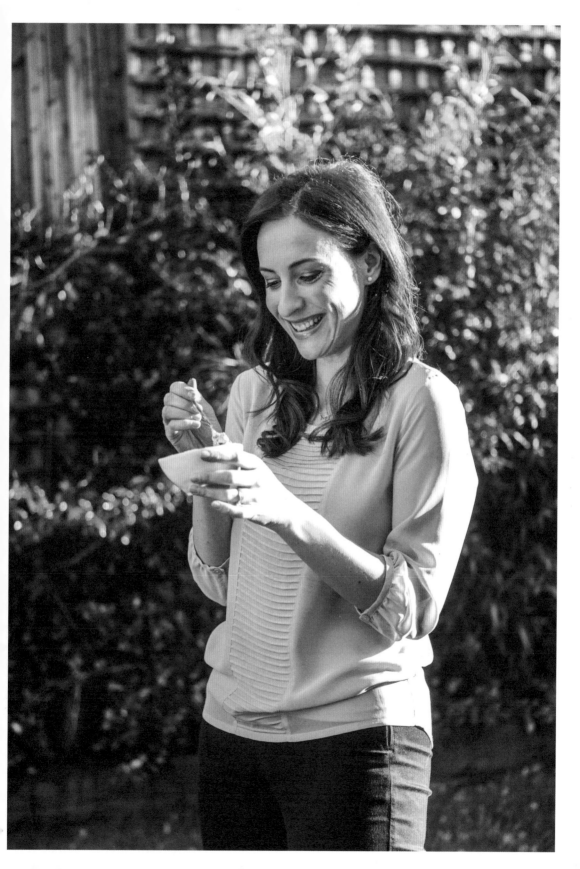

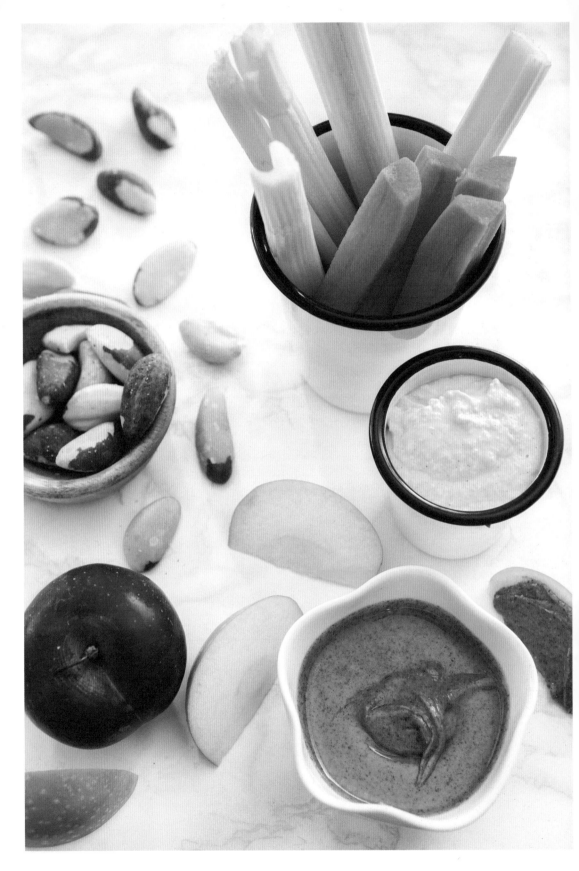

SIDES, DIPS AND SNACKS

Simple Cauliflower Mash

1 small head of cauliflower, trimmed and cut into small florets
1 tablespoon olive oil or butter
1/3 cup finely grated Parmesan cheese (optional)
salt and freshly ground black pepper

Serves 4

Puréed or mashed cauliflower makes a wonderful substitute for mashed potato. Low in carbs but high in nutrients, you'll be surprised at just how mild and delicious this healthy mash tastes. You can flavour it up in a multitude of ways, but I've kept this version nice and simple.

1 Bring a large pot of salted water to a boil. Add the cauliflower and cook for 10–15 minutes, until very tender. Reserve ¼ cup of the cooking liquid, then drain well and transfer the cauliflower to a food processor (alternatively, you can use a potato masher).

2 Add the oil or butter and the reserved water 1 tablespoon at a time and purée or mash until smooth. Stir in the Parmesan (if using) and season with salt and pepper.

Classic Hummus

It can be hard to find a shop-bought hummus that you really love. If you have a food processor or blender, you can whip up a hummus that's exactly to your taste in a matter of minutes. I like to dip strips of crunchy red pepper into my hummus for a scrumptious snack.

1 x 400g can chickpeas, rinsed and drained
1 garlic clove, minced
3 tablespoons fresh lemon juice
2 tablespoons olive oil
2 tablespoons tahini
2 tablespoons water
1 teaspoon sea salt
½ teaspoon paprika (optional)
pinch of freshly ground black pepper

Makes 4–6 servings

1 Place all the ingredients into a food processor and whizz until smooth. Spoon into a serving dish and refrigerate until ready to use.
2 Serve with salad and strips of whole wheat pitta bread for lunch or pair with crunchy veggie sticks or oatcakes for a filling and satisfying snack.

Quinoa

1 cup quinoa

2 cups water

1 heaped teaspoon
   vegetable bouillon
   powder or stock of your
   choice

Makes approx. 6 servings

Quinoa (pronounced keen-wa) is a super seed that originates from Peru. Try eating it in place of rice, pasta or couscous. As well as being delicious, it packs a serious nutritional punch because it's high in protein, B vitamins and minerals such as iron and magnesium. Quinoa works well served hot as part of a meal or soup or cold in salads.

1   Rinse the quinoa in a sieve under a running tap. Put into a saucepan and add the water and bouillon. Bring to the boil and simmer with the lid on for 15 minutes. Allow to sit, covered, for 5 minutes more after cooking. Stir with a fork. It will have absorbed all the remaining water and should be light and fluffy.

Simple Guacamole

Anything that tastes delicious and makes my skin glow at the same time is a real winner in my book, and avocados do just that. The healthy fats and vitamins in avocados moisturise and nourish your skin from the inside out. I swear I see a difference in my skin when I eat them.

**2 ripe avocados, peeled and
   sliced**
1 ripe tomato, chopped
**¼ small onion, finely
   chopped**
1 garlic clove, minced
**juice of ½–1 lime (depending
   on taste; I use 1 lime)**
**salt and freshly ground
   black pepper**

Serves 6

1 Place the avocados in a medium serving bowl and mash with a fork until you reach your desired consistency. Sir in the chopped tomato, onion and garlic. Add lime juice and seasoning to taste and mix well.
2 If you like your guacamole super smooth, use a blender instead. To enhance the flavours, chill the guacamole for half an hour before serving.

Super Simple Salad Dressings

You can transform a salad from drab to fab with a simple dressing. Make your favourite salad dressing and store it in the fridge in a sealed container such as a jam jar. That way you always have a delicious dressing on hand to jazz up your salads and veggies.

CLASSIC FRENCH DRESSING
6 tablespoons extra virgin
  olive oil
2 tablespoons white wine
  vinegar
1 teaspoon Dijon mustard
½ small garlic clove, minced
pinch of sea salt and freshly
  ground black pepper

**SIMPLE LEMON AND OIL
VINAIGRETTE**
6 tablespoons extra virgin
  olive oil
juice of 1 lemon
pinch of sea salt and freshly
  ground black pepper

BALSAMIC DRESSING
6 tablespoons extra virgin
  olive oil
2 tablespoons balsamic
  vinegar (choose a brand
  with no added sugar)
pinch of sea salt and freshly
  ground black pepper

1 Put all the ingredients into an empty jam jar. Screw the lid on tightly and give it a good shake, then season with salt and pepper to taste. Store in the fridge and use as needed. Make sure to always re-shake before use to blend the ingredients together again.

Oats-So-Healthy Brown Bread

What makes this brown bread different is that it's free from wheat flour and yeast, which is great for anyone who is sensitive to or bloats from eating standard bread. Oats are high in a type of fibre called beta-glucan, which helps to lower cholesterol and improve blood sugar control. Don't be put off by the ingredients list – this bread is so moist and delicious, you won't want to go back to ordinary bread, especially when you realise just how quick and easy it is to make.

300g oats
2 tablespoons sesame seeds
2 teaspoons bread soda
pinch of salt
500g whole milk natural yoghurt (not low-fat)

Makes 1 loaf

1 Preheat the oven to 175°C. Grease a 1lb loaf tin.
2 Place the oats, seeds, bread soda and a pinch of salt into a large bowl. Pour over the yoghurt and mix the ingredients together really well. Pour the mixture evenly into the greased tin. The mixture should take up about three-quarters of the volume of the tin. Smooth the top with the back of a spoon to ensure it's nice and even.
3 Bake in the oven for approximately 50 minutes. Use a skewer to check that it's cooked through. If you feel it's going quite brown on top, just cover it loosely with a little tin foil for the last 10 minutes.
4 Once baked, let it cool in the tin for at least 10 minutes, then remove to a wire rack to cool completely.

Variations
There are lots of things you can add to this recipe, including cinnamon, mixed spice, mixed seeds or nuts, black olives or rosemary to name but a few. Experiment with whatever tickles your fancy.

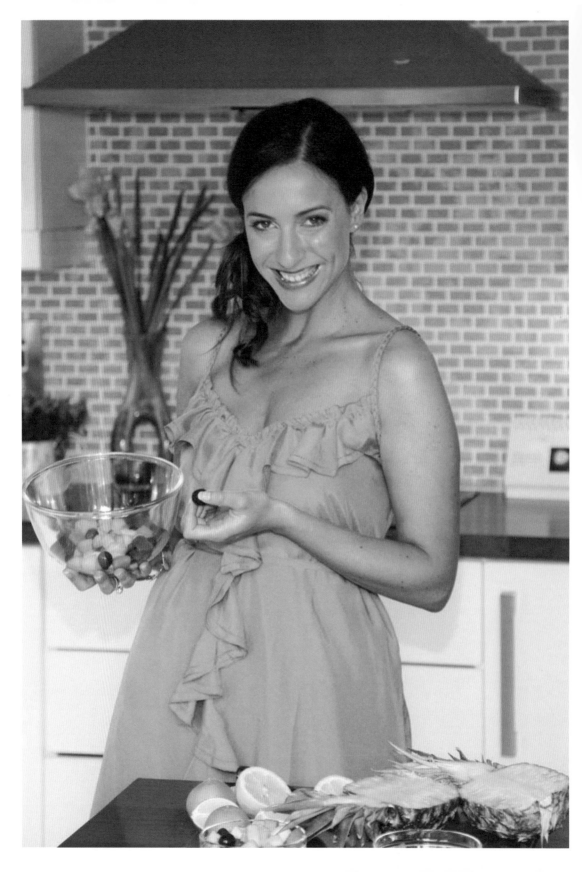

SWEET-ISH TREATS

Comforting Apple and Strawberry Crumble

800g cooking apples,
   peeled, cored and sliced
200g strawberries,
   quartered
3 tablespoons water
pinch of salt
1 cup rolled oats
½ cup chopped almonds
   (ideally chopped in a
   food processor)
1 teaspoon ground
   cinnamon
1 large tablespoon coconut
   oil, melted
natural Greek yoghurt or
   fresh cream, to serve

Serves 4–6

This mouth-watering crumble is naturally sweet and very versatile, as any combination of fruit can be used. It's also super quick and easy to make and yes, you guessed it, it's sugar-free!

1   Preheat the oven to 190°C.
2   Place the fruit into a baking dish, then add the water and toss with a pinch of salt to bring out some of the natural sweetness in the fruit.
3   In a separate bowl, mix together the oats, almonds and cinnamon, then pour in the melted coconut oil and mix well. Spoon the crumble mixture over the fruit to cover it entirely.
4   Bake the crumble for 30–35 minutes, until the fruit is tender and bubbling. Serve this not-so-naughty dessert with a dollop of natural Greek yoghurt or fresh cream.

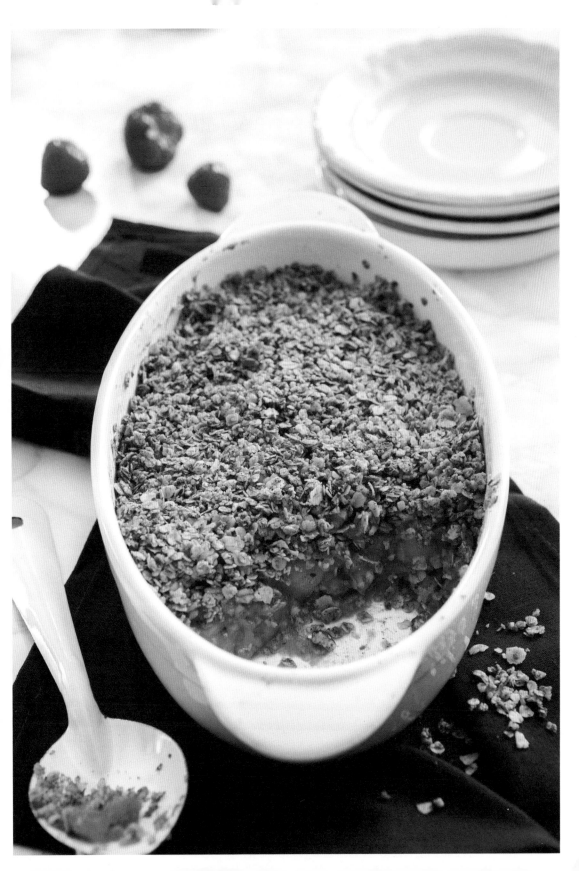

Banana Walnut Bread

3 medium ripe bananas,
  mashed
50g butter, at room tem-
  perature
½ cup (125ml) natural Greek
  yoghurt
2 eggs, beaten
275g self-raising whole
  wheat flour
1 heaped teaspoon ground
  cinnamon
½ cup chopped walnuts

Makes 1 loaf

This is a healthy version of banana bread.
It's denser and less sweet than most other
recipes, but still tastes great. I love making
this for an occasional treat and the house
smells amazing after baking it.

The extra protein and fibre in this recipe
help to balance out the sugars from the
bananas so it won't spike your blood sugar –
provided you stick to one slice!

1   Preheat the oven to 180°C. Lightly grease
    a 1lb loaf tin.
2   In a large bowl, combine the mashed
    bananas, butter, yoghurt and beaten
    eggs. Beat well and set aside.
3   Place the flour and cinnamon in a
    separate bowl and stir well. Add the
    dry ingredients to the mashed banana
    mixture, beating until blended. Stir in the
    nuts.
4   Spoon the batter into the greased tin.
    Bake for 60 minutes, until a knife inserted
    in the middle comes out dry. Cool in the tin
    for 10 minutes, then turn out and cool on a
    wire rack for a further 20 minutes.

Banana and Peanut Butter Cookies

The beauty of these cookies is that they can be made up and baked in less than 30 minutes using only four simple ingredients. They taste more cakey than crunchy, almost like mini banana breads. The oats and bananas form the basis for these cookies, but after that you could add any combination of nuts, seeds or spices that you like. Personally, I like the simplicity of flavours in this recipe.

2 ripe bananas
1 cup rolled oats
½ cup peanuts, chopped
1 heaped tablespoon peanut butter

Makes 8–10 cookies

1 Preheat the oven to 180°C. Line a baking tray with parchment paper.
2 In a medium bowl, mash the bananas really well with a fork until no lumps remain. Stir in the oats until well blended and let the mixture stand for 5 minutes. Stir in the chopped peanuts and the peanut butter. (You can chop the peanuts with a knife or in a food processor.)
3 Drop the mixture onto the lined baking tray 1 tablespoon at a time. Flatten a bit using a rubber spatula.
4 Bake in the oven for 12–15 minutes, until lightly golden. Cool on a wire rack and store in an airtight container for a few days. They keep for up to five days in the fridge.

Mood-Lifting Chocolate Mousse

1 cup whole milk Greek yoghurt, at room temperature
140g dark chocolate (minimum 70% cocoa solids)
½ cup whole milk
½ teaspoon vanilla extract
pinch of salt (optional)
1 teaspoon grated dark chocolate, to decorate

Serves 2–4

If nothing but chocolate will do, then this dark chocolate mousse should hit the spot. Dark chocolate does contain sugar, but considerably less than milk chocolate so it can be enjoyed in small quantities as an occasional treat. The protein and fat from the Greek yoghurt will help slow down the absorption of sugars from the chocolate. Rich, creamy and somewhat indulgent, this is a real mood-lifting mousse.

1 Pour the Greek yoghurt into a large bowl, draining off any excess liquid first. Set aside.

2 Bring a pot of water to a gentle boil, and place a glass bowl snugly on top of the pot – but don't allow the bowl to be immersed in or touch the water. Add the milk, vanilla extract and salt to the bowl and heat, whisking frequently, over a medium heat until hot but not boiling.

3 Break the chocolate into small, even-sized pieces and add to the milk. Let it sit for 1 minute in the heated milk without touching it, then gently stir with a spatula until the chocolate melts into the milk. Remove from the heat and continue stirring slowly until it's completely smooth.

4 Whip the yoghurt with a fork until it's fluffy. Stir the chocolate mixture again, then gently fold it into the yoghurt bit by bit using a spatula until it's fully combined. This takes about 2 minutes.

5 Divide the mixture into individual ramekins, small bowls or shot glasses. Sprinkle a little grated dark chocolate on top if desired. Chill for at least 2 hours before serving cold.

Healthy Energy Bars

If you need an energy boost, these snack bars are just the ticket. The banana adds a touch of sweetness but the protein and fat from the nuts and seeds will ensure you get a nice slow steady release of energy. These are perfect to ward off on afternoon slump.

3 medium bananas
1 teaspoon pure vanilla extract
2 cups rolled oats
½ cup walnuts, chopped
½ cup chopped or flaked almonds
½ cup sunflower or hemp seeds
½ cup pumpkin seeds
1 teaspoon ground cinnamon
¼ teaspoon fine sea salt

Makes 12–14 bars

1 Preheat the oven to 180°C. Lightly grease a large rectangular baking tray and line with a piece of parchment paper so the bars lift out easily.

2 Mash the bananas in a large bowl until smooth. Stir in the vanilla, then add the oats and combine well. Add the walnuts and almonds and combine well, followed by the seeds, cinnamon and salt. Mix until thoroughly combined.

3 Spoon the mixture onto the prepared baking tray. Press down with the back of a spoon until compacted and smooth out with your hands until it's even.

4 Bake for approx. 25 minutes, until firm and lightly golden around the edges. Place the baking tray on a cooling rack for 10 minutes, then carefully slide a knife around the edges to loosen the ends and lift out the slab. Place the slab on a wire cooling rack for approx 20 minutes. Slice into small 10cm x 10cm bars and store in an airtight container.

Index